*A*lthough there is no cure for diabetes, for most people the diabetes treatment program will include a healthy diet, exercise and medication. An important element in any diabetes treatment is proper nutrition. We have increased the print size to make the recipes easier to read, and marked all the low carbohydrate recipes with this special icon for your convenience:

We hope with these improvements, these quick and easy recipes will be a useful tool for the diabetic and low carbohydrate dieter or anyone who wants to improve their diet.

With Our Love,

Linda and Emily

Linda Coffee and Emily Cale

Copyright 2003

PLEASE NOTE THE FOLLOWING ABOUT THE NUTRIENT ANALYSIS OF THE RECIPES IN THE DIABETIC FOUR INGREDIENT COOKBOOK:

The analysis for the cookbook was done using the Nutritionist IV Diet and Recipe Analysis and Nutrition Evaluation (N-Squared Incorporated 1993) computer software program which includes the USDA database of foods and an All Foods database. Additional foods were added to the database by using manufacturer's food labels.

Recipes can be further modified to decrease sodium and fat by omitting salt and reducing the oil, margarine or fat from the recipe or by using unsalted or fat-free products when available.

A recipe that has 400mg or more of sodium per serving is considered a high sodium food as per the American Diabetes Association and the American Dietetic Association. A recipe that contains 10 grams or less of carbohydrates per serving is considered a low carbohydrate food.

Recipe analysis is an approximation and different results may be obtained by using different nutrient databases. Manufacturer's nutrition labels may also change affecting the nutrient content of the recipe.

Information about Exchange Lists and Carbohydrates:

Exchange lists are foods listed together because they are alike. Each serving of food has about the same amount of carbohydrate, protein, fat and calories as the other food on that list. That is why any food on a list can be "exchanged" or traded for any other food on the same list. For example, you can trade the slice of bread you might eat for breakfast for 1/2 cup of cooked cereal. Each of these foods equals one starch choice.

The Exchange List lists foods with their serving sizes, which are usually measured after cooking. When you begin, you should measure the size of each serving. This may help you learn to "eyeball" correct serving sizes.

The Exchange List provides you with a lot of food choices and gives you a variety in your meals and recipes. Several foods, such as dried beans and peas, bacon, and peanut butter are in 2 categories. This gives you flexibility in putting your meals together. Whenever you choose new foods or vary your meal plan, monitor your blood glucose to see how these different foods affect your blood glucose level.

Fitting Sugar In Your Meal Plan

It is commonly thought that people with diabetes should avoid all forms of sugar. Most people with diabetes can eat foods containing sugar as long as the total amount of carbohydrate from that meal or snack is consistent and sugar foods are added within the context of healthy eating. Many research studies have shown that meals which contain sugar do not make the blood sugar rise higher than meals of equal carbohydrate levels which do not contain sugar. However, if the sugar-containing meal contains more carbohydrates, the blood sugar levels will go up.

For example: Which will have the greater effect on blood sugar?
_____1 tsp. sugar or _____1/2 cup potatoes

The potatoes will contribute about 15 grams of carbohydrates, while a level teaspoon of sugar will only give 4 grams of carbohydrates. Therefore, the potatoes will have about three times the effect on blood sugar as compared to the table sugar.

It is important to realize that sugar is not the only carbohydrate that you have to control. The body will convert all carbohydrates to glucose – so eating extra servings of rice, pasta, bread, fruit or other carbohydrates foods will make the blood sugar rise.

DIETARY CHANGES YOU CAN DO
TO REDUCE FAT AND SUGAR FROM YOUR MEALS

1. Eat more chicken, fish and turkey.
2. Eat red meat only three (3) times a week.
3. Choose lean cuts of meat - for beef cuts, look for 'loin' or 'round' in the name of the meat. Pork tenderloin is a leaner cut of meat. Chicken breast is also leaner than dark meat like the thighs and legs.
4. Trim visible fat from meat before cooking.
5. Skin the chicken and remove visible fat beneath the skin before cooking.
6. Limit red meat, chicken and fish to 6 ounces a day.
7. Choose cheese that is fat free or made from part skim milk or low fat milk.
8. Choose lunchmeats that are at least 99% fat free.
9. Drink milk, that has no more than 1% fat. Fat free milk is best.
10. Limit oils, fats, egg yolks, organ meats, sour cream, bacon, sausage, gravies, lard, butter and cheese.
11. Limit cakes pies, cookies, butter crackers and sweet bread.
12. No more fried foods - bake, grill, broil or boil your meats instead.
13. Eat 3 meals a day and do not skip meals.
14. Eat smaller portions - cut your normal portion in half and add a salad - you will save a lot of calories.
15. Drink diet soda - regular soda has about 15 teaspoons of sugar per can.
16. Use sugar substitute instead of sugar.
17. Eat fresh fruit with the peel instead of desserts.
18. Eat 100% whole wheat bread instead of white bread, for more fiber.
19. Eat raw vegetables all day.
20. Do not drink juice - eat fresh fruit with the peel instead (has more fiber and less sugar).

NEW LOW FAT WAYS TO COOK

Instead Of:	Try This:
Whole Milk	Fat Free Milk
Cream	Evaporated Fat Free Milk
Buttered Bread Crumbs	Crushed Corn Flakes/Crackers
Flour and Fat (for thickening)	Cornstarch and Water
Sour Cream	Plain Fat Free Yogurt
Butter, Lard, Shortening and Other Solid Fats	Soft Tub Margarine, Canola Oil, Safflower Oil or Sunflower Oil
Cheddar or Swiss Cheese	Part Skim Mozzarella or Fat Free Cheese
Whole Egg (yolk and white)	2 Egg Whites or Egg Substitutes
Bacon	Canadian Bacon
Sirloin or Chuck	Round or Flank Steak
Ground Beef	Lean Ground Turkey
Lunchmeat or Hotdogs	Lean Ham or Turkey Breast 99% Fat Free
Cheese Enchiladas	Chicken Enchiladas
Sauteed Vegetables	Steamed Vegetables
Refried Beans	Boiled Beans with Cilantro and Spices - No Bacon Added
Ice Cream	Non-Fat Desserts or Fat Free Frozen Yogurt Sweetened with Aspartame

Here is a list of a few helpful foods that you will want to keep on hand as you become a low fat, sugar-free cook. This is also a good list to check before you head off to the grocery store so that you will have everything you need to make healthy, satisfying meals!

DAIRY PRODUCTS:
Fat Free Milk
Fat Free Yogurt made/Aspartame
Non Fat Dry Milk
Part Skim Mozzarella
Part Skim Ricotta
Low Fat Swiss Cheese

MEAT & PROTEIN:
Chicken Breasts
Water Packed Tuna
Super Lean Ground Beef
Lean Ground Turkey
Round Steak
Lean Pork Loin
Fish Fillets (Cod, Flounder, Red Snapper or Orange Roughy)

STARCH / BREAD:
100% Whole Wheat Bread
Brown Rice
White Rice
Bran Muffin Mix
(made with water, not oil)
Fresh Potatoes
Corn Tortillas
Low Fat Whole Wheat Crackers
Low Fat High Fiber Cereal
(Fiber One, All Bran)
Dried Beans
(pinto, kidney, navy, lentils)
Rolled Oats

EXTRA/ DESSERTS/SNACKS:
Sugar Free Gelatin
Angel Food Cake
Sugar Free, Fat Free Pudding
Ginger Snaps
Graham Crackers
Pretzels
Animal Crackers
Air Popped Popcorn
Natural Flavor Microwave
Popcorn

FRUITS & VEGETABLES:
Fresh or Frozen Vegetables
Carrots
Green Beans
Cauliflower
Lettuce/Greens (Spinach/Red Leaf)
Tomatoes
Cucumbers
Onions
Yellow Squash
Zucchini
Apples
Oranges
Peaches
Pears
Plums
Grapefruit

SEASONINGS:
Lemon Juice
Salt Free Seasoning
Butter Substitute
Sugar Substitute
Salsa
Horseradish
Garlic Powder
Black Pepper / Crushed Red Pepper
Rosemary
Vinegar
Fat Free Salad Dressing
Fat Free Margarine
Canola Oil
Olive Oil
Nonstick Spray
Fresh Garlic and Fresh Herbs

LOW FAT AND LOW SUGAR SNACK LIST

Here are a few healthy but tasty snacks that you and your family can enjoy. The correct portion size is listed and the diabetic exchange it counts as:

CRUNCHY SNACKS:

88 Pretzel Sticks . . . . .1 Starch
16 Pretzel Chips (Mr. Phipps brand) . . . . .1 Starch
3 Cups Air Popped or Plain Microwave Popcorn . . . . .1 Starch
10 Baked Tortilla Chips . . . . .1 Starch
5 Mini-Rice Cakes or 2 Rice Cakes (4-inches) . . . . .1 Starch
6 Saltine Crackers . . . . .1 Starch
1 Cup Dry Cheerios . . . . .1 Starch
2 Hard Breadsticks . . . . .1 Starch
4 Slices of Melba Toast . . . . .1 Starch
24 Oyster Crackers . . . . .1 Starch
5 Fat Free Whole Wheat Crackers . . . . .1 Starch
1 Cup Raw Carrots or Raw Vegetables . . . . .1 Vegetable

SWEET SNACKS:

3 Graham Cracker Squares . . . . .1 Starch
8 Animal Crackers . . . . .1 Starch
3 Gingersnap Cookies . . . . .1 Starch
2 Fig Cookies (small) . . . . .1 Starch
18 Teddy Graham Snacks . . . . .1 Starch
1/2 Cup Frozen Sugar Free Nonfat Yogurt . . . . .1 Milk
1 Cup Light Nonfat Yogurt Made with Aspartame . . . . .1 Milk
1/2 Cup Sugar Free Pudding . . . . .1 Milk
1 Cup Fresh Fruit . . . . .1 Fruit
1/2 Cup Water or Juice Packed Canned Fruit . . . . .1 Fruit
5 Vanilla Wafers . . . . .1 Starch and 1 Fat
1 Oatmeal Cookie . . . . .1 Starch and 1 Fat

If you suspect you may have diabetes, ask yourself these few simple questions. If you answer yes to more than 2 and have more than 2 of the signs and symptoms, you will want to see your family physician for a complete check-up as soon as possible.

	YES	NO
1. Are you overweight?	☐	☐
2. Are you over 30 years old?	☐	☐
3. Do you have family history of diabetes?	☐	☐
4. Have you had two or more fasting blood sugars over 126?	☐	☐
5. Are you physically inactive?	☐	☐
6. Are you African American, Native American or Hispanic?	☐	☐
7. Are you a woman who has had a baby weighing 9 pounds or more at birth?	☐	☐
8. Do you have any of these signs or symptoms:		
Extreme Thirst?	☐	☐
Frequent Urination?	☐	☐
Blurry Vision?	☐	☐
Fatigue/Drowsiness?	☐	☐
Unexplained Weight Loss?	☐	☐

VERY IMPORTANT

BY ANSWERING THESE QUESTIONS WITH A "YES" IT IS NOT A DIAGNOSIS OF DIABETES. YOU MUST TALK TO YOUR DOCTOR FIRST.

TABLE OF CONTENTS

APPETIZERS 1

SALADS 55

VEGETABLES 101

MAIN DISHES

    CHICKEN 157

    FISH 205

    PORK 243

    BEEF 269

PASTA 299

SAUCES 311

DESSERTS 327

Appetizers

SHRIMP SPREAD

1. **2 Cans (4 1/2 oz. each) Shrimp (drained)**
2. **2 Cups Fat Free Mayonnaise**
3. **6 Green Onions (chopped fine)**
4. **Whole Wheat Low Sodium Crackers**

Crumble shrimp. Mix first three ingredients and refrigerate for at least one hour. Serve with crackers.

SERVING SIZE - 2 CRACKERS & 1 TEASPOON SPREAD

Calories	79	Protein	4g
Total Fat	0g	Carbohydrate	17g
Saturated Fat	0g	Cholesterol	12mg
Sodium	243mg	Fiber	6g

EXCHANGES: 1 Bread

ITALIAN SHRIMP DIP

1. 1 Carton (8 oz.) Fat Free Sour Cream
2. 1 Package (8 oz.) Fat Free Cream Cheese (softened)
3. 1 Package Italian Salad Dressing Mix
4. 1 Can (4 oz.) Shrimp (drained, finely chopped)

Mix above ingredients and chill. Serve on celery sticks. 6 Servings.

PER SERVING – 1/3 CUP

Calories	88	Protein	17g
Total Fat	0g	Carbohydrate	5g
Saturated Fat	0g	Cholesterol	42mg
Sodium	526mg	Fiber	0g

EXCHANGES: 2 1/2 Meat, 1/2 Milk

EASY CRAB SPREAD

1. **1 Package (8 oz.) Fat Free Cream Cheese**
2. **1 Bottle (12 oz.) Cocktail Sauce**
3. **1 Can (6 oz.) Crab Meat (drained)**

Spread cream cheese on dinner plate and pour bottle of cocktail sauce over cream cheese. Crumble crab meat on top of the cocktail sauce. Serve with low fat crackers. 8 Servings.

PER SERVING – 1/3 CUP

Calories	102	Protein	10g
Total Fat	1g	Carbohydrate	12g
Saturated Fat	0g	Cholesterol	26mg
Sodium	809mg	Fiber	0g

EXCHANGES: 1 1/2 Meats, 1 Starch

HOT SEAFOOD DIP

1. 2 (8 oz. each) Packages Fat Free Cream Cheese
2. 1/2 Cup Fat Free Milk
3. 1 Tablespoons Worcestershire Sauce
4. 1 Can (6 1/2 oz.) Crab Meat

Soften cream cheese to room temperature. Mix all ingredients. Bake 15 minutes at 350 degrees. Serve with fresh vegetables. 8 Servings.

PER SERVING – 1/4 CUP

Calories	91	Protein	17g
Total Fat	1g	Carbohydrate	5g
Saturated Fat	0g	Cholesterol	33mg
Sodium	546mg	Fiber	0g

EXCHANGES: 2 1/2 Lean Meats, 1/2 Milk

JALAPENO PIE

1. 1 Can (11 oz.) Jalapeno Peppers
2. 3/4 Cup Egg Beaters
3. 2 Cups Grated Fat Free Cheddar Cheese
4. Salt And Pepper (optional)

Seed, rinse and slice peppers. Place peppers in greased 9-inch pie plate sprayed with cooking spray. Sprinkle cheese over peppers. Pour seasoned eggs over cheese. Bake 20 minutes at 400 degrees. Cut into small slices and serve.

SERVING SIZE - 1/16 OF PIE

Calories	50	Protein	10g
Total Fat	0g	Carbohydrate	1g
Saturated Fat	0g	Cholesterol	5mg
Sodium	503mg	Fiber	0g

EXCHANGES: 1 1/2 Very Lean Meats

GREEN CHILI PIE

1. 1 Can (4.5 oz) Diced Green Chilies
2. 2 Cups Fat Free Mozzarella Cheese
3. 1 Container (4 oz.) Egg Beaters (equal 2 eggs)
4. 1 Green Onions (chopped)

Place green chilies in a 7 1/2x11 1/2-inch oven proof casserole. Sprinkle with cheese and onions. Pour eggs over top. Sprinkle with paprika for garnish. Bake at 350 degrees for 10-15 minutes. 15 Servings.

PER SERVING - 1/15 OF PIE

Calories	48	Protein	10g
Total Fat	0g	Carbohydrate	2g
Saturated Fat	0g	Cholesterol	5mg
Sodium	292mg	Fiber	0g

EXCHANGES: 1 1/2 Lean Meats, 1/2 Vegetable

COTTAGE CHEESE-CUCUMBER SPREAD

1. 1 Cup Cucumber (finely chopped)
2. 1 Cup Small Curd Fat Free Cottage Cheese
3. Dash Pepper
4. Minced Chives

Mix cucumber, cottage cheese and pepper. Spread on lowfat whole wheat crackers and garnish with minced chives.

SERVING SIZE - PER TEASPOON

Calories	4	Protein	1g
Total Fat	0g	Carbohydrate	0g
Saturated Fat	0g	Cholesterol	0mg
Sodium	20mg	Fiber	0g

EXCHANGES: Free food up to 7 tsp. (8 tsp. = 1 Very Lean Meat)

HAM AND PIMIENTO SPREAD

LOW CARB

1. 1 1/2 Cups Extra Lean Cooked Ham (finely chopped)
2. 1 Jar (4 oz.) Pimiento (drained, chopped)
3. 1/2 Cup Fresh Parsley (chopped)
4. 1/2 Cup Fat Free Mayonnaise

Mix all ingredients and stir well. Chill. Serve on celery sticks or melba toast. 8 Servings.

PER SERVING – 1/3 CUP

Calories	59	Protein	6g
Total Fat	2g	Carbohydrate	5g
Saturated Fat	1g	Cholesterol	14mg
Sodium	518mg	Fiber	0g

EXCHANGES: 1 Very Lean Meat, 1/2 Starch

STUFFED MUSHROOMS

1. **1 Pound Mushrooms (half dollar size)**
2. **1 Cup Bread Crumbs**
3. **2 Tablespoons Fat Free Margarine**
4. **2 Slices Fat Free Ham Lunch Meat (chopped)**

Remove stems and inside of mushrooms. Chop stems and mix with remaining ingredients. Stuff mushrooms and place in Pam-sprayed casserole dish. Bake 15 minutes at 350 degrees.

SERVING SIZE - PER MUSHROOM

Calories	43	Protein	2g
Total Fat	1g	Carbohydrate	7g
Saturated Fat	0g	Cholesterol	2mg
Sodium	116mg	Fiber	0g

EXCHANGES: 1/2 Bread

PARTY RYE BREAD

1. **1 Package Party Rye Bread**
2. **1 Cup Fat Free Mayonnaise**
3. **3/4 Cup Fresh Parmesan Cheese**
4. **1 Green Onion Bunch (chopped fine)**

Mix mayonnaise, cheese and onion. Spread on bread and broil 2-3 minutes.

SERVING SIZE - 4 SLICES PARTY RYE BREAD &
1 TEASPOON SPREAD

Calories	127	Protein	6g
Total Fat	4g	Carbohydrate	17g
Saturated Fat	0g	Cholesterol	7mg
Sodium	547mg	Fiber	0g

EXCHANGES: 1 Bread, 1 Lean Meat

HOT ARTICHOKE SPREAD

1. 1 Cup Fat Free Mayonnaise
2. 1 Cup Freshly Grated Parmesan Cheese
3. 1 Can (4 oz.) Green Chilies (chopped)
4. 1 Cup Of Canned Artichoke Hearts (chopped)

Mix mayonnaise, parmesan cheese, green chiles and artichoke hearts. Put 1 teaspoon of the mixture on bite-size lowfat toast rounds. Broil until lightly brown.

SERVING SIZE - PER TEASPOON

Calories	49	Protein	4g
Total Fat	2g	Carbohydrate	3g
Saturated Fat	0g	Cholesterol	6mg
Sodium	270mg	Fiber	0g

EXCHANGES: 1/2 Vegetable, 1/2 Very Lean Meat, 1/2 Fat

SPANISH OLIVE SPREAD

1. 1 Carton (8 ounces) Fat Free Sour Cream
2. 1/4 Cup Green Pimiento Stuffed Olives (chopped)
3. 1/4 Cup Liquid From Olive Jar
4. Paprika

In blender place sour cream and olive liquid and blend until smooth. Pour into bowl and add olives. Mix thoroughly. Sprinkle with paprika and refrigerate. Serve as a spread on party rye bread. 4 Servings.

PER SERVING – 1/3 CUP

Calories	58	Protein	7g
Total Fat	4g	Carbohydrate	3g
Saturated Fat	0g	Cholesterol	0mg
Sodium	603mg	Fiber	1g

EXCHANGES: 1 Meat

PIMIENTO CHEESE SPREAD I

1. 2 Cups Fat Free Cottage Cheese
2. 1 Teaspoon Onion Powder
3. 1 Jar (3 oz.) Pimientos (drained)

Mix above ingredients in blender. Serve as a spread or stuff celery sticks. 6 Servings.

PER SERVING – 1/3 CUP

Calories	51	Protein	9g
Total Fat	0g	Carbohydrate	4g
Saturated Fat	0g	Cholesterol	3mg
Sodium	283mg	Fiber	0g

EXCHANGES: 1 1/2 Meat

PIMIENTO CHEESE SPREAD II

1. **1 Pound Fat Free Cheese (grated)**
2. **1 Jar (3 oz.) Pimientos (drained)**
3. **1/2 Cup Fat Free Mayonnaise**

Blend above ingredients until smooth. Spread on crackers or vegetables. 6 Servings.

PER SERVING – 1/3 CUP

Calories	128	Protein	24g
Total Fat	0g	Carbohydrate	7g
Saturated Fat	0g	Cholesterol	14mg
Sodium	796mg	Fiber	0g

EXCHANGES: 1/2 Starch, 3 1/2 Meat

SAN ANTONE BEAN DIP

1. 1 Can (10 1/4 oz.) Condensed Black Bean Soup
2. 1 Can (8 oz.) Tomato Sauce
3. 1 Cup Fat Free Sour Cream
4. 1/2 Teaspoon Chili Powder

Heat all ingredients in sauce pan. Stir mixture occasionally. Serve with fat free baked tortilla chips.

SERVING SIZE - PER TABLESPOON

Calories	6	Protein	1g
Total Fat	0g	Carbohydrate	1g
Saturated Fat	0g	Cholesterol	0mg
Sodium	62mg	Fiber	0g

EXCHANGES: Free up to 5 tbsp.
(6 tsp. = 1/2 Bread, 1/2 Very Lean Meat)

MINI QUICHES

1. 1 Can Refrigerator Lowfat Biscuits
2. 1 Cup Lowfat Low Sodium Monterey Jack (shredded)
3. 1/2 Cup Egg Beaters
4. 2 Green Onions With Tops (finely chopped)

Separate rolls and divide each roll into three sections. Press dough section in lightly greased mini-muffin cups stretching slightly to form shell. Mix cheese, eggs and onions and spoon mixture into shells. Bake for 15 minutes or until firm at 375 degrees.

SERVING SIZE - PER MINI QUICHE

Calories	40	Protein	3g
Total Fat	2g	Carbohydrate	4g
Saturated Fat	1g	Cholesterol	4mg
Sodium	127mg	Fiber	0g

EXCHANGES: 2 Mini Quiches = 1/2 Bread, 1 Lean Meat

PINEAPPLE BALL

1. 1 Package (8 oz.) Fat Free Cream Cheese
2. 1 Can (3 1/2 oz.) Water Packed Crushed
   Pineapple (drained)
3. 2 Tablespoons Green Pepper (chopped)
4. 1 Teaspoon Lawry's Seasoned Salt

Mix cream cheese, pineapple, green pepper and sprinkle with Lawry's Seasoned Salt. Shape into a ball and serve with lowfat crackers.

SERVING SIZE - PER TABLESPOON

Calories	18	Protein	3g
Total Fat	0g	Carbohydrate	2g
Saturated Fat	0g	Cholesterol	3mg
Sodium	235mg	Fiber	0g

EXCHANGES: 3 Tablespoons = 1/2 Bread

FRESH STRAWBERRY DIP

1. 3 Cups Fresh Strawberries
2. 1 Cup Fat Free Sour Cream
3. 1 Tablespoon Brown Sugar
4. 1/2 Teaspoon Vanilla

Mix sour cream and brown sugar. Serve with strawberries. 4 Servings.

PER SERVING – 1/4 CUP

Calories	78	Protein	7g
Total Fat	0g	Carbohydrate	13g
Saturated Fat	0g	Cholesterol	0mg
Sodium	33mg	Fiber	2g

EXCHANGES: 1 Meat, 1 Fruit

ALMOND DELIGHT DIP

1. **2 Cartons (8 oz. each) Vanilla Non Fat Yogurt**
2. **1/8 Teaspoon Almond Extract**
3. **2 Tablespoons Chopped Toasted Almonds**

Combine yogurt and almond extract. Chill at least 1 hour. Sprinkle with chopped almonds. Serve with assorted fresh fruit. 4 Servings.

PER SERVING – 1/4 CUP

Calories	165	Protein	9g
Total Fat	6g	Carbohydrate	21g
Saturated Fat	0g	Cholesterol	2mg
Sodium	70mg	Fiber	1g

EXCHANGES: 1 Milk, 1 Starch, 1 Fat

CARAMEL FRUIT DIP

1. **1 Package (8 oz.) Fat Free Cream Cheese (softened)**
2. **1/2 Cup Brown Sugar**
3. **1 Teaspoon Vanilla**
4. **1 Cup Fat Free Sour Cream**

Mix above ingredients and chill. Serve with assorted fresh fruit. 4 Servings.

PER SERVING – 1/2 CUP

Calories	198	Protein	18g
Total Fat	0g	Carbohydrate	33g
Saturated Fat	0g	Cholesterol	10mg
Sodium	446mg	Fiber	0g

EXCHANGES: 2 1/ 2 Meat, 1/2 Milk, 2 Starch

ALMOND FRUIT DIP

1. **2 Cups (16 oz.) Fat Free Cottage Cheese**
2. **1/2 Cup Powdered Sugar**
3. **1 Package (4 oz.) Fat Free Cream Cheese**
4. **1 Teaspoon Almond Extract**

In blender, add above ingredients and blend until smooth. Cover and chill until ready to serve. Serve with fresh fruit. 6 Servings.

PER SERVING – 1/2 CUP

Calories	103	Protein	13g
Total Fat	0g	Carbohydrate	13g
Saturated Fat	0g	Cholesterol	7mg
Sodium	415mg	Fiber	0g

EXCHANGES: 2 Meat, 1 Starch

APPLE CURRY DIP

1. **1 1/2 Cups Fat Free Cottage Cheese**
2. **1 Cup Unsweetened Applesauce**
3. **1 Envelope Onion Soup Mix**
4. **2 Teaspoons Curry Powder**

In blender, blend cottage cheese and applesauce until smooth. Stir in soup mix and curry powder. Serve with fresh vegetables. 4 Servings.

PER SERVING – 1/2 CUP

Calories	83	Protein	10g
Total Fat	0g	Carbohydrate	11g
Saturated Fat	0g	Cholesterol	4mg
Sodium	329mg	Fiber	1g

EXCHANGES: 1 1/2 Meat, 3/4 Fruit

FRUITED CHEESE SPREAD

1. **1 Package (8 oz.) Fat Free Cream Cheese (room temperature)**
2. **1 Tablespoon Concentrated Orange Juice (defrosted)**
3. **Few Drops Vanilla**
4. **1/2 Cup Mandarin Oranges (chopped)**

Combine above ingredients and mix well. Spread on toast rounds or slices of high fiber bread cut in fourths. 8 Servings

PER SERVING – 1/4 CUP

Calories	41	Protein	6g
Total Fat	0g	Carbohydrate	4g
Saturated Fat	0g	Cholesterol	5mg
Sodium	203mg	Fiber	0g

EXCHANGES: 1 Lean Meat, 1/2 Fruit

TROPICAL CHEESE SPREAD

1. **1/2 Cup Fat Free Cheese**
2. **1/4 Cup Crushed Pineapple (drained)**
3. **1 Teaspoon Lemon Juice**

Combine ingredients and mix in blender until smooth. Serve on melba toast. 2 Servings.

PER SERVING – 1/3 CUP

Calories	45	Protein	7g
Total Fat	0g	Carbohydrate	5g
Saturated Fat	0g	Cholesterol	3mg
Sodium	211mg	Fiber	0g

EXCHANGES: 1 Meat

CHILI CON QUESO

1. **2 Pounds Fat Free Velveeta Cheese (grated)**
2. **1 Can (10 oz.) Rotel Tomatoes and Green Chilies**

Melt cheese slowly in saucepan or microwave. Stir in tomatoes. Use as a dip with fat free tortilla chips or fresh vegetables.

SERVING SIZE - PER TABLESPOON

Calories	17	Protein	4g
Total Fat	0g	Carbohydrates	1g
Saturated Fat	0g	Cholesterol	1mg
Sodium	94mg	Fiber	0g

EXCHANGES: 1/2 Meat

CHILE SALSA

1. **1 Cup Chopped Seeded Tomatoes**
2. **1/2 Cup Chopped Green Onions**
3. **1 Can (4 oz.) Diced Green Chiles**

Mix above ingredients together and refrigerate.
Serve with fresh vegetables or fat free tortilla chips.
4 Servings.

PER SERVING – 1/2 CUP

Calories	22	Protein	1g
Total Fat	0g	Carbohydrate	5g
Saturated Fat	0g	Cholesterol	0mg
Sodium	356mg	Fiber	1g

EXCHANGES: 1 Vegetable

MEXICAN AVOCADO DIP

1. 3 Large Ripe Avocados (mashed)
2. 1 Cup Fat Free Sour Cream
3. 1 Package Good Season Mexican Salad Dressing Mix
4. 1 Tablespoon Lemon Juice

Mix above ingredients or process in food processor until smooth. Serve with fat free tortilla chips.
6 Servings.

PER SERVING – 1/3 CUP

Calories	177	Protein	6g
Total Fat	15g	Carbohydrate	9g
Saturated Fat	2g	Cholesterol	0mg
Sodium	233mg	Fiber	3g

EXCHANGES: 3 Fats, 1 Meat, 1/2 Starch

MEXICAN MEATBALLS

1. **1 Pound Extra Lean Ground Beef**
2. **1 Package Taco Seasoning Mix**
3. **Salsa**

Mix lean ground beef and taco seasoning and shape into 1-inch meatballs. Brown in skillet and place on paper towel to drain. Reheat in oven and serve with chilled salsa. 25 Meatballs.

SERVING SIZE - PER MEATBALL

Calories	57	Protein	4g
Total Fat	4g	Carbohydrate	1g
Saturated Fat	2g	Cholesterol	14mg
Sodium	44mg	Fiber	0g

EXCHANGES: 1/2 Very Lean Meat, 1 Fat

SHERRIED MEATBALLS

1. **2 Pounds Extra Lean Ground Beef**
2. **1 Cup Catsup**
3. **1 Cup Cooking Sherry**
4. **2 Tablespoons Brown Sugar**

Heat oven to 350 degrees. Season ground beef to taste and shape into 1-inch meatballs. Place meatballs in oven for 30 minutes to brown. Remove meatballs from browning pan and place into a casserole. Mix remaining three ingredients and pour over meatballs. Bake an additional 30 minutes. Serve meatballs with sauce. 50 Meatballs.

PER SERVING - PER MEATBALL

Calories	56	Protein	3g
Total Fat	3g	Carbohydrate	2g
Saturated Fat	1g	Cholesterol	12mg
Sodium	77mg	Fiber	0g

EXCHANGES: 1/2 Meat, 1/2 Fat

PARTY DRUMMETTES

1. **2 Pounds Chicken Drummettes (skin removed)**
2. **1/4 Cup Low Sodium Soy Sauce**
3. **1/4 Cup Wine Vinegar**
4. **1/4 Teaspoon Garlic Powder**

Broil drummettes, 8 minutes one side, turn and broil 6 minutes on other side until browned. Combine drummettes with remaining ingredients in a shallow baking dish. Cover and bake at 350 degrees for 30 minutes or until done. Makes 20 drummettes.

PER SERVING - 1 DRUMMETTE

Calories	110	Protein	8g
Total Fat	8g	Carbohydrate	0g
Saturated Fat	2g	Cholesterol	37mg
Sodium	153mg	Fiber	0g

EXCHANGES: 1 Fat, 1 Meat

CALIFORNIA DIP

1. 2 Cups Fat Free Cottage Cheese
2. 1 Tablespoon Lemon Juice
3. 2 Tablespoons Skim Milk
4. 1 Envelope Dry Onion Soup Mix

Mix cottage cheese and lemon juice in blender Add skim milk. Place in bowl and stir in onion soup mix. Chill before serving with fresh vegetables.

SERVING SIZE - PER TABLESPOON

Calories	7	Protein	1g
Total Fat	0g	Carbohydrates	0g
Saturated Fat	0g	Cholesterol	0mg
Sodium	41mg	Fiber	0g

EXCHANGES: Free Food for 1 Tbsp. (4 Tbsp. = 1 Vegetable)

COTTAGE CHEESE DIP

1. **1 Carton (24 oz.) Fat Free Cottage Cheese**
2. **1 Envelope Herb Ox Dry Broth Mix**
3. **1/3 Cup Fat Free Milk**

Blend all ingredients, chill and serve with fresh vegetables. 6 Servings.

PER SERVING – 1/2 CUP

Calories	75	Protein	13g
Total Fat	0g	Carbohydrate	5g
Saturated Fat	0g	Cholesterol	5mg
Sodium	431mg	Fiber	0g

EXCHANGES: 2 Meats

DILL DIP

1. 1 Carton (12 oz.) Fat Free Cottage Cheese
2. 2 1/2 Teaspoons Dill
3. 1/4 Teaspoons Seasoned Salt
4. 2 Tablespoons Lemon Juice

Combine all ingredients in blender. Blend at low speed. Refrigerate several hours for better flavor. Sprinkle with additional dill and serve with fresh vegetables. 4 Servings.

PER SERVING – 1/3 CUP

Calories	56	Protein	10g
Total Fat	0g	Carbohydrate	4g
Saturated Fat	0g	Cholesterol	4mg
Sodium	452mg	Fiber	0g

EXCHANGES: 1 1/2 Meat

CREAMY DILL DIP

1. **1 Cup Fat Free Miracle Whip**
2. **2 Tablespoons Onion (finely chopped)**
3. **1 Tablespoon Fat Free Milk**
4. **1 Teaspoon Dill**

Mix all ingredients and chill. Serve with fresh vegetables. 4 Servings.

PER SERVING – 1/3 CUP

Calories	84	Protein	0g
Total Fat	0g	Carbohydrate	21g
Saturated Fat	0g	Cholesterol	0mg
Sodium	843mg	Fiber	0g

EXCHANGES: 1 1/2 Bread

CREAM CHEESE DIP

1. 1 Package (8 oz.) Fat Free Cream Cheese
2. 1 1/2 Tablespoons Lemon Juice
3. 1 1/2 Teaspoons Onion (grated)
4. 2 Cups Fat Free Sour Cream

Let cream cheese soften at room temperature. Cream until smooth. Add lemon juice and onion; blend well. Gradually blend sour cream. Chill. Serve with fresh vegetables. 6 Servings.

PER SERVING – 1/2 CUP

Calories	82	Protein	16g
Total Fat	0g	Carbohydrate	6g
Saturated Fat	0g	Cholesterol	7mg
Sodium	311mg	Fiber	0g

EXCHANGES: 1/2 Milk, 2 1/2 Meat

SPRING VEGETABLE DIP

1. **1 Envelope Dry Vegetable Soup Mix**
2. **2 Cups Fat Free Sour Cream**

Combine soup mix and sour cream. Refrigerate for two hours or overnight before serving. Serve with fresh vegetables. 4 Servings.

PER SERVING – 1/2 CUP

Calories	62	Protein	12g
Total Fat	0g	Carbohydrate	4g
Saturated Fat	0g	Cholesterol	0mg
Sodium	73mg	Fiber	0g

EXCHANGES: 1 1/2 Meat

SOUR CREAM DIP

1. **1 Cup Fat Free Sour Cream**
2. **1/2 Tablespoon Prepared Mustard**
3. **2 Tablespoons Chili Sauce**
4. **1/4 Teaspoon Celery Seed**

Combine all ingredients. Chill. Serve with celery sticks and cucumber slices. 4 Servings.

PER SERVING – 1/3 CUP

Calories	41	Protein	6g
Total Fat	0g	Carbohydrate	4g
Saturated Fat	0g	Cholesterol	0mg
Sodium	155mg	Fiber	0g

EXCHANGES: 1 Meat

AVOCADO AND LEEK DIP

1. 1 Large Ripe Avocado (mashed)
2. 1 Tablespoon Fresh Lemon Juice
3. 1/2 Package Dry Leek Soup Mix
4. 1 Cup Fat Free Sour Cream

Mix mashed avocado with lemon juice. Combine with soup mix and sour cream. Serve with fresh vegetables. 4 Servings.

PER SERVING – 1/3 CUP

Calories	108	Protein	7g
Total Fat	8g	Carbohydrate	5g
Saturated Fat	1g	Cholesterol	0mg
Sodium	42mg	Fiber	2g

EXCHANGES: 1 Meat, 1 1/2 Fat

TOMATO-SOUR CREAM DIP

1. 1 Can (8 oz.) Tomato Sauce
2. 1 Cup Fat Free Sour Cream
3. 2 Teaspoons Grated Onion
4. 1 Teaspoon Horseradish

Combine all ingredients. Chill. Serve with fresh vegetables. 4 Servings.

PER SERVING – 1/2 CUP

Calories	50	Protein	7g
Total Fat	0g	Carbohydrate	7g
Saturated Fat	0g	Cholesterol	0mg
Sodium	402mg	Fiber	1g

EXCHANGES: 1 Meat, 1/2 Starch

ARTICHOKE RANCH DIP

1. 1 Can (8 1/2 oz.) Artichoke Hearts (drained and finely chopped)
2. 1 Tablespoon Light Ranch Salad Dressing Mix
3. 1 Package (8 oz.) Fat Free Cream Cheese (softened)
4. 1 Cup Fat Free Mayonnaise

Mix above ingredients and refrigerate. Serve with fresh vegetables. 6 Servings.

PER SERVING – 1/2 CUP

Calories	106	Protein	9g
Total Fat	0g	Carbohydrate	18g
Saturated Fat	0g	Cholesterol	7mg
Sodium	1130mg	Fiber	2g

EXCHANGES: 1 Meat, 1/2 Milk, 1 Vegetable, 1/2 Starch

TANGY DIP

1. **1 Cup Fat Free Sour Cream**
2. **2 Tablespoons Chili Sauce**
3. **2 Teaspoons Prepared Horseradish**

Mix above ingredients. Cover and refrigerate at least one hour. Serve with fresh vegetables. 4 Servings.

PER SERVING – 1/3 CUP

Calories	39	Protein	6g
Total Fat	0g	Carbohydrate	4g
Saturated Fat	0g	Cholesterol	0mg
Sodium	133mg	Fiber	0g

EXCHANGES: 1 Meat

CURRY DIP

1. 1 Cup Fat Free Sour Cream
2. 1 Teaspoon Curry Powder
3. 1/2 Teaspoon Lemon Juice
4. 1/2 Teaspoon Ground Cumin

Combine above ingredients and chill. Serve with fresh vegetables. 4 Servings.

PER SERVING – 1/3 CUP

Calories	33	Protein	6g
Total Fat	0g	Carbohydrate	2g
Saturated Fat	0g	Cholesterol	0mg
Sodium	31mg	Fiber	0g

EXCHANGES: 1 Meat

ROQUEFORT DIP

1. 1/2 Cup Crumbled Bleu Cheese
2. 2 Cups Fat Free Cottage Cheese
3. 1 Teaspoon Dried Onion Flakes
4. Pepper to Taste

Combine and blend above ingredients. Chill until ready to serve. Serve with fresh vegetables.
6 Servings.

PER SERVING –1/3 CUP

Calories	88	Protein	11g
Total Fat	3g	Carbohydrate	3g
Saturated Fat	2g	Cholesterol	12mg
Sodium	437mg	Fiber	0g

EXCHANGES: 1/2 Fat, 1 1/2 Meat

POTATO SKINS

1. **4 Potatoes (baked)**
2. **8 Ounces Reduced Fat Cheddar Cheese (grated)**
3. **1 Cup Fat Free Sour Cream**
4. **2 Tablespoons Chopped Green Onion**

Cut each potato into quarters lengthwise. Scoop out pulp. Spray potato skins with cooking spray and place on baking pan. Bake at 425 degrees for 10 minutes. Turn and bake for an additional 5-8 minutes or until crisp and light brown. Remove from oven and place cheese, sour cream and onions on each quarter. Return to oven and bake until cheese melts.

SERVING SIZE - PER QUARTER

Calories	103	Protein	7g
Total Fat	3g	Carbohydrates	14g
Saturated Fat	2g	Cholesterol	10mg
Sodium	123mg	Fiber	1g

EXCHANGES: 1 Bread, 1 Lean Meat

HIDDEN VALLEY RANCH CHEESE PUFFS

1. 2 Cups Fat Free Shredded Sharp Cheddar Cheese
2. 3/4 Cup Fat Free Mayonnaise
3. 1 Tablespoon Hidden Valley Ranch Milk Mix
4. 10 (1-inch) Slices French Bread

Mix first three ingredients. Spread on bread slices. Broil until golden brown (about 3 minutes).
10 Servings.

PER SERVING – 1 SLICE BREAD

Calories	132	Protein	9g
Total Fat	1g	Carbohydrate	20g
Saturated Fat	0g	Cholesterol	0mg
Sodium	762mg	Fiber	0g

EXCHANGES: 1 Starch, 1/2 Meat, 1/2 Milk

VEGGIE DIPPIN' DIP

1. 1 Package (8 oz.) Fat Free Herb/Garlic Cream
   Cheese (softened)
2. 2 Tablespoons Skim Milk
3. 1 Teaspoon Prepared Horseradish
4. 1/2 Cup Parsley

Mix above ingredients and beat until smooth. Serve
with raw vegetables.

SERVING SIZE - PER TABLESPOON

Calories	11	Protein	2g
Total Fat	0g	Carbohydrates	1g
Saturated Fat	0g	Cholesterol	2mg
Sodium	71mg	Fiber	0g

EXCHANGES: 3 Tablespoons - 1 Very Lean Meat

TORTILLA ROLLUPS

1. **1 Package (8 oz.) Fat Free Cream Cheese (softened)**
2. **1 Teaspoon Taco Seasoning**
3. **1/3 Cup Picante Sauce**
4. **12 Flour Tortillas**

Beat cream cheese until smooth. Add taco seasoning, picante sauce and mix well. Spread mixture on each tortilla. Roll tortilla tightly. Place seam side down in airtight container. Chill at least two hours. Slice each roll into 1 inch slices forming a pinwheel. Arrange on plate to serve.

SERVING SIZE - PER PINWHEEL

Calories	23	Protein	1g
Total Fat	0g	Carbohydrates	4g
Saturated Fat	0g	Cholesterol	1mg
Sodium	62mg	Fiber	0g

EXCHANGES: 4 Pinwheels = 1 Bread

CRAB DELIGHT

1. **2 Packages (8 oz. each) Fat Free Cream Cheese (softened)**
2. **1 Package (8 oz.) Imitation Crab Meat**
3. **2 Tablespoons Green Onions (finely chopped)**
4. **1/2 Cup Bottled Horseradish Sauce**

Beat cream cheese until smooth and blend in remaining ingredients. Spread into pie plate. Bake uncovered for 20 minutes at 375 degrees. Serve with lowfat crackers or vegetables.

SERVING SIZE - PER TABLESPOON

Calories	18	Protein	3g
Total Fat	0g	Carbohydrates	2g
Saturated Fat	0g	Cholesterol	3mg
Sodium	154mg	Fiber	0g

EXCHANGES: 2 Tablespoons - 1 Very Lean Meat

LIGHT GUACAMOLE

1. **1 Bag (20 oz.) Frozen Peas (defrosted)**
2. **1/4 Cup Fresh Lime Juice**
3. **1/2 Bunch of Green Onions (diced)**
4. **1/4 Cup Picante Sauce**

In blender, blend peas, lime juice and onions. Remove to mixing bowl and mix in picante sauce. Refrigerate until ready to serve. Serve with fat free tortilla chips.

SERVING SIZE - PER TABLESPOON

Calories	10	Protein	1g
Total Fat	0g	Carbohydrates	2g
Saturated Fat	0g	Cholesterol	0mg
Sodium	20mg	Fiber	0g

EXCHANGES: Free up to 2 Tablespoons (3 Tbsp. = 1/2 Bread)

PIZZA CRACKERS

1. **4 Dozen Melba Or Cracker Rounds**
2. **3/4 Cup Ketchup**
3. **2 Ounces Thinly Sliced Pepperoni**
4. **1 Cup Shredded Lowfat, Low Sodium Mozzarella Cheese**

Spread rounds with ketchup and top with pepperoni slices. Sprinkle with cheese and bake on cookie sheet 3 to 5 minutes at 400 degrees.

SERVING SIZE - PER CRACKER

Calories	41	Protein	2g
Total Fat	2g	Carbohydrates	3g
Saturated Fat	1g	Cholesterol	3mg
Sodium	106mg	Fiber	0g

EXCHANGES: 3 Crackers = 1/2 Bread, 1 Medium Fat Meat

HOMEMADE FAT FREE TORTILLA CHIPS

1. **Corn Tortillas**
2. **1/4 Teaspoon Cumin**
3. **1/4 Teaspoon Pepper**
4. **1/4 Teaspoon Salt**

Cut stack of tortillas into 8 wedges each. Spread wedges in a single layer on a baking sheet. Sprinkle with cumin, pepper and salt (optional). Bake at 375 degrees about 10 minutes or until dry and crisp. Monitor chips as to not overbrown. Turn after 5 minutes. Store in air-tight container. When serving, freshen up in microwave about one minute. Let sit about 5 minutes before serving or they will be soft and chewy.

SERVING SIZE - 20 CHIPS

Calories	140	Protein	4g
Total Fat	2g	Carbohydrates	29g
Saturated Fat	0g	Cholesterol	0mg
Sodium	157mg	Fiber	0g

EXCHANGES: 2 Breads

BAGEL CHIPS

1. **Lowfat Bagel**
2. **No Fat Butter Flavored Spray**
3. **1/8 Teaspoon Garlic Powder**
4. **1/8 Teaspoon Cajun Seasoning**

Slice bagel into 1/4-inch thick rounds. Place in microwave bowl and cook on high for one minute. Gently stir. Continue to microwave in one minute increments, stirring after each minute, approximately 3 minutes. Watch carefully. Chips should be crisp. (If over-microwaved char spots will appear.) Remove from microwave and spray with butter flavored spray and sprinkle with garlic and cajun seasoning. 2 Servings.

SERVING SIZE- 1/2 OF CHIPS

Calories	104	Protein	4g
Total Fat	19	Carbohydrate	20g
Saturated Fat	09	Cholesterol	0mg
Sodium	195 mg	Fiber	0g

EXCHANGES: 1 1/2 Starches

Salads

MARINATED VEGETABLE SALAD

1. **2 Cups Cauliflower Pieces**
2. **2 Cups Broccoli Pieces**
3. **1 Basket Cherry Tomatoes (cut in halves)**
4. **1 Bottle (8 oz.) Fat Free Italian Dressing**

Mix above ingredients and chill overnight.
6 Servings.

SERVING SIZE - PER CUP

Calories	45	Protein	2g
Total Fat	0g	Carbohydrate	9g
Saturated Fat	0g	Cholesterol	0mg
Sodium	553mg	Fiber	2g

EXCHANGES: 2 Vegetables

LUNCHEON TUNA SALAD

1. **1 Can (10 oz.) Water Packed Tuna (drained)**
2. **1 Can (8 oz.) Low Sodium Peas (drained)**
3. **3/4 Cup Celery (finely chopped)**
4. **1/2 Cup Fat Free Mayonnaise**

Toss all ingredients and chill. Serve on a bed of lettuce. 4 Servings.

SERVING SIZE - 3/4 CUP

Calories	151	Protein	20g
Total Fat	2g	Carbohydrate	16g
Saturated Fat	0g	Cholesterol	13mg
Sodium	460mg	Fiber	3g

EXCHANGES: 1 Bread, 2 1/2 Very Lean Meat

SWEET POTATO SALAD

1. 3 Sweet Potatoes (approximately 1/2 lb. each)
2. 1 Medium Onion (sliced into thin rings)
3. 1 Green Pepper (cut into thin strips)
4. 1/4 Cup Fat Free Vinaigrette Dressing

Heat enough water to boiling to cover sweet potatoes. Add sweet potatoes and return to boil. Cover and cook 30 minutes or just until fork tender. Do not overcook. Cool and slice into 1/4-inch slices. Combine sweet potato slices, onion rings and green pepper strips in large bowl. Refrigerate at least one hour. Toss lightly with vinaigrette dressing.
8 Servings.

SERVING SIZE - 1/2 CUP

Calories	81	Protein	1g
Total Fat	0g	Carbohydrate	19g
Saturated Fat	0g	Cholesterol	0mg
Sodium	112mg	Fiber	3g

EXCHANGES: 1 Bread

APPLE COLESLAW

1. **2 Cups Cabbage (shredded)**
2. **2 Medium Apples (cored, diced)**
3. **1 Can (16 oz.) Crushed Pineapple (drained)**
4. **3/4 Cup Fat Free Mayonnaise**

Combine above ingredients, cover and refrigerate 1 hour or more before serving. 8 Servings.

SERVING SIZE - 3/4 CUP

Calories	60	Protein	1g
Total Fat	0g	Carbohydrate	15g
Saturated Fat	0g	Cholesterol	0mg
Sodium	257mg	Fiber	2g

EXCHANGES: 1/2 Bread, 1/2 Fruit

BELL PEPPER SALAD

1. 1 Medium Red Bell Pepper (sliced)
2. 1 Medium Green Bell Pepper (sliced)
3. 1 Medium Yellow Bell Pepper (sliced)
4. 1/4 Cup Fat Free Italian Dressing

Mix peppers in large bowl and toss with dressing. Refrigerate until ready to serve. 6 Servings.

SERVING SIZE - 3/4 CUP

Calories	50	Protein	2g
Total Fat	0g	Carbohydrate	2g
Saturated Fat	0g	Cholesterol	0mg
Sodium	143mg	Fiber	2g

EXCHANGES: 1 1/2 Vegetables, 1/2 Bread

HEARTS OF PALM SALAD

1. 6 Cups Boston Lettuce (torn in bite-sized pieces)
2. 6 Green Onions (sliced)
3. 1 Can (14 oz.) Hearts of Palm (drained, sliced horizontally)
4. 1/2 Cup Fat Free Wine Vinaigrette Dressing

Toss lettuce, onions and hearts of palm. Pour over salad and serve with vinaigrette dressing.
6 Servings.

PER SERVING – 1 CUP

Calories	52	Protein	3g
Total Fat	0g	Carbohydrate	11g
Saturated Fat	0g	Cholesterol	0mg
Sodium	321mg	Fiber	4g

EXCHANGES: 2 Vegetables

SNOW PEA SALAD

1. **2 Cups Snow Peas (trimmed)**
2. **1 Red Bell Pepper (sliced)**
3. **1 Teaspoon Toasted Sesame Seeds**
4. **1/2 Cup Hidden Valley Fat Free Italian Parmesan Salad Dressing**

Blanch the snow peas and drain, running under cold water. Pat dry and refrigerate for an hour. When ready to serve, place snow peas in a circle on individual plates. Arrange red pepper strips between snow peas and sprinkle with sesame seeds. Drizzle salad dressing over top of each salad. 6 Servings.

PER SERVING – 1/2 CUP

Calories	143	Protein	7g
Total Fat	5g	Carbohydrate	17g
Saturated Fat	1g	Cholesterol	9mg
Sodium	531mg	Fiber	4g

EXCHANGES: 3 Vegetable, 1 Fat

ITALIAN TOMATO CHEESE SALAD

1. 12 Cherry Tomatoes (cut in halves)
2. 1 Ounce Fat Free Mozzarella Cheese (cut in cubes)
3. 4 Pitted Black Olives (sliced)
4. 1 Tablespoon Fat Free Italian Salad Dressing

Mix above ingredients and toss lightly to coat with dressing. Refrigerate until chilled. Serve on a bed of lettuce. 4 Servings.

PER SERVING – 1/2 CUP

Calories	29	Protein	3g
Total Fat	1g	Carbohydrate	3g
Saturated Fat	0g	Cholesterol	1mg
Sodium	146mg	Fiber	1g

EXCHANGES: 1/2 Very Lean Meat, 1/2 Vegetable

CUCUMBER STRAWBERRY SALAD

1. **1/4 Cup Fresh Lime Juice**
2. **1 Small Green Pepper (diced)**
3. **1 Cucumber (peeled, sliced)**
4. **2 Cups Fresh Strawberries (quartered)**

Combine lime juice and pepper. Toss mixture with cucumbers and strawberries. Chill before serving. 4 Servings.

SERVING SIZE - 1 CUP

Calories	49	Protein	1g
Total Fat	0g	Carbohydrate	12g
Saturated Fat	0g	Cholesterol	0mg
Sodium	3mg	Fiber	3g

EXCHANGES: 1/2 Vegetable, 1/2 Fruit

CARROT SALAD

1. 2 Cups Grated Carrots
2. 1/2 Cup Raisins
3. 1 Can (8 3/4 oz.) Water Packed Pineapple Tidbits (drained)
4. 1/3 Cup Low Fat Mayonnaise

Combine above ingredients and serve on a crisp bed of lettuce. 6 Servings.

SERVING SIZE - 1/2 CUP

Calories	117	Protein	1g
Total Fat	4g	Carbohydrate	22g
Saturated Fat	0g	Cholesterol	0mg
Sodium	126mg	Fiber	3g

EXCHANGES: 1 1/2 Vegetable, 1 Fruit, 1/2 Fat

CARROT RAISIN CELERY SALAD

1. **6 Cups Carrots (grated)**
2. **1 Cup Raisins**
3. **2 Cups Celery (sliced)**
4. **1/3 Cup Fat Free Mayonnaise**

Mix above ingredients and chill at least 1 hour.
8 Servings.

PER SERVING – 1 CUP

Calories	166	Protein	3g
Total Fat	0g	Carbohydrate	41g
Saturated Fat	0g	Cholesterol	0mg
Sodium	210mg	Fiber	6g

EXCHANGES: 3 1/2 Vegetables, 1 1/2 Fruits

PASTA SALAD

1. **1 Package (16 oz.) Elbow Macaroni Pasta (cooked, rinsed, drained)**
2. **1 Medium Sweet Red Pepper (cut into strips)**
3. **1 Cup Fresh Mushrooms (sliced)**
4. **1 Cup Broccoli Flowerets**

Combine ingredients and toss well. Chill and serve with fat free salad dressing of your choice.
8 Servings.

SERVING SIZE - 1/2 CUP

Calories	88	Protein	3g
Total Fat	0g	Carbohydrate	18g
Saturated Fat	0g	Cholesterol	0mg
Sodium	4mg	Fiber	2g

EXCHANGES: 1/2 Vegetable, 1 Bread

SEAFOOD PASTA SALAD

1. 1 Pound Vegetable Rotini Pasta (cooked, rinsed, drained)
2. 1 Package (10 oz.) Frozen Chopped Broccoli (thawed, drained)
3. 1 Package (8 oz.) Imitation Crab Flakes
4. 1/2 Cup Fat Free Italian Dressing

Combine pasta with ingredients. Toss and chill until ready to serve. Garnish with finely chopped green onions. 6 Servings.

PER SERVING – 3/4 CUP

Calories	157	Protein	9g
Total Fat	1g	Carbohydrate	28g
Saturated Fat	0g	Cholesterol	8mg
Sodium	614mg	Fiber	5g

EXCHANGES: 1/2 Vegetable, 1 1/2 Starch, 1/2 Very Lean Meat

ORANGE SALAD

1. 1 Can (8 oz.) Water Packed Crushed Pineapple (drained)
2. 1 Package (3 oz.) Sugar Free Orange Jello
3. 1 Carton (12 oz.) Small Curd Fat Free Cottage Cheese
4. 1 Carton (8 oz.) Lite Cool Whip

Mix pineapple, orange jello, cottage cheese. Fold in Cool Whip and chill until ready to serve. 8 Servings.

SERVING SIZE - 1/2 CUP

Calories	99	Protein	5g
Total Fat	4g	Carbohydrate	11g
Saturated Fat	0g	Cholesterol	3mg
Sodium	185mg	Fiber	0g

EXCHANGES: 1/2 Very Lean Meat, 1 1/2 Fat

SEAFOOD SALAD

1. **1 Package (8 oz.) Crab Delights (flake style)**
2. **1/2 Cup Lowfat Mayonnaise**
3. **2 Stalks Celery (chopped)**
4. **3 Tablespoons Onion (finely chopped)**

Combine ingredients. Serve on a crisp bed of lettuce.
4 Servings.

SERVING SIZE - 1/2 CUP

Calories	148	Protein	7g
Total Fat	8g	Carbohydrate	11g
Saturated Fat	1g	Cholesterol	11mg
Sodium	715mg	Fiber	0g

EXCHANGES: 1 Very Lean Meat, 1 1/2 Fat

TURKEY SALAD

1. **3 Cups Cooked Cubed Turkey Breasts**
2. **1 Can (16 oz.) Pineapple Tidbits (drained)**
3. **1 Can (8 oz.) Sliced Water Chestnuts (drained)**
4. **4 Green Onions (sliced)**

Combine above ingredients and serve with a fat free honey mustard dressing. Nutrient breakdown does not include salad dressing. 6 Servings.

PER SERVING –1 CUP

Calories	197	Protein	35g
Total Fat	1g	Carbohydrate	11g
Saturated Fat	0g	Cholesterol	95mg
Sodium	63mg	Fiber	1g

EXCHANGES: 1 Vegetable, 1/2 Fruit, 5 Very Lean Meats

SPINACH CHICKEN SALAD

1. 2 Packages (10 oz.) Frozen Chopped Spinach
2. 1 Pound Chicken Breasts (cooked, skinless, boneless)
3. 2 Tablespoons Lemon Pepper
4. 1 Cup Fat Free Mayonnaise

Thaw spinach and pat dry with paper towel. Place in large bowl. Shred chicken breasts and add to spinach. Toss spinach and chicken with lemon pepper and mayonnaise. 6 Servings.

PER SERVING – 3/4 CUP

Calories	218	Protein	20g
Total Fat	10g	Carbohydrate	14g
Saturated Fat	1g	Cholesterol	38mg
Sodium	633mg	Fiber	3g

EXCHANGES: 1 Vegetable, 2 1/2 Very Lean Meats, 1/2 Fat, 1/2 Starch

GREEN BEAN SALAD

1. 1 Can (16 oz.) French Style Green Beans (drained)
2. 8 Cherry Tomatoes (halved)
3. 4 Fresh Green Onions (sliced)
4. 1/2 Cup Fat Free French Dressing

Combine ingredients. Chill at least one hour before serving. Serve on a crisp bed of lettuce. 4 Servings.

SERVING SIZE - 1/2 CUP

Calories	77	Protein	2g
Total Fat	0g	Carbohydrate	16g
Saturated Fat	0g	Cholesterol	0mg
Sodium	531mg	Fiber	2g

EXCHANGES: 1 1/2 Vegetables, 1/2 Bread

BEET AND ONION SALAD

1. 1/4 Cup Wine Vinegar
2. 1 Packet Equal (or sugar substitute)
3. 1 Can (16 oz.) Sliced Beets (undrained)
4. 1/2 Onion (sliced in rings)

Combine above ingredients and marinate at room temperature at least 30 minutes before serving. Stir every 10 minutes. 4 Servings.

PER SERVING – 1/2 CUP

Calories	56	Protein	2g
Total Fat	0g	Carbohydrate	14g
Saturated Fat	0g	Cholesterol	0mg
Sodium	302mg	Fiber	0g

EXCHANGES: 1 Starch

BROCCOLI SALAD

1. 2 Cups Fresh Broccoli (cut into bite-sized pieces)
2. 2 Ounces Feta Cheese (crumbled)
3. 1/2 Head Lettuce (torn in bite-sized pieces)
4. 1/2 Cup Fat Free Italian Dressing

Combine above ingredients and serve. 6 Servings.

PER SERVING – 1/2 CUP

Calories	44	Protein	3g
Total Fat	2g	Carbohydrate	4g
Saturated Fat	1g	Cholesterol	8mg
Sodium	410mg	Fiber	1g

EXCHANGES: 1/2 Vegetable, 1/2 Fat

MARINATED CAULIFLOWER SALAD

1. 2 Cups Cauliflower (divided into flowers and thinly sliced)
2. 1 Small Onion (thinly sliced)
3. 12 Small Pimiento-stuffed Olives (sliced)
4. 1/3 Cup Kraft Fat Free Catalina Salad Dressing

Mix all ingredients, cover and refrigerate at least 1 hour before serving. Stir occasionally. 4 Servings.

PER SERVING   1/2 CUP

Calories	56	Protein	2g
Total Fat	2g	Carbohydrate	10g
Saturated Fat	0g	Cholesterol	0mg
Sodium	416mg	Fiber	0g

EXCHANGES: 1 Vegetable

CORN SALAD

1. **2 Cans (16 oz.) Mexicorn (drained)**
2. **1 Green Pepper (chopped)**
3. **1 Onion (chopped)**
4. **1 Cup Kraft Fat Free Italian Salad Dressing**

Combine ingredients. Chill several hours. Serve cold.
4 Servings.

PER SERVING - 1 CUP

Calories	257	Protein	16g
Total Fat	1g	Carbohydrate	59g
Saturated Fat	0g	Cholesterol	0mg
Sodium	1269mg	Fiber	6g

EXCHANGES: 1 Vegetable, 3 1/2 Starches

CUCUMBER SALAD

1. **2 Cups Cucumbers (peeled and sliced)**
2. **2 Onions (sliced)**
3. **1 Packet Equal or Sugar Substitute**
4. **1 Cup Fat Free Sour Cream**

Place cucumbers and onions in bowl. Sprinkle with sugar substitute. Add sour cream and mix. Salt and pepper to taste. Refrigerate for several hours. 6 Servings.

PER SERVING – 1/2 CUP

Calories	44	Protein	5g
Total Fat	0g	Carbohydrate	6g
Saturated Fat	0g	Cholesterol	0mg
Sodium	49mg	Fiber	1g

EXCHANGES: 1 Vegetable, 1/2 Very Lean Meat

HONEY CUCUMBER SALAD

1. 1/4 Cup White Vinegar
2. 1 Tablespoon Honey
3. 1/2 Medium Green Pepper (diced)
4. 2 Cups Cucumbers (peeled, thinly sliced)

Combine vinegar and honey and pour over cucumbers and green peppers. Chill for several hours before serving. 4 Servings.

PER SERVING – 1/2 CUP

Calories	32	Protein	0g
Total Fat	0g	Carbohydrate	8g
Saturated Fat	0g	Cholesterol	0mg
Sodium	2mg	Fiber	0g

EXCHANGES: 1 Vegetable

SWEET AND SOUR CUCUMBER SALAD

1. 2 Cup Cucumbers (peeled, sliced)
2. 1/2 Teaspoon Salt
3. 1 Tablespoon Vinegar
4. 3 Tablespoons Sugar

Place sliced cucumbers in bowl and mix well with salt. Let stand 15 minutes. Drain off all the salty fluid. Add vinegar and sugar and let stand 10 minutes. Before serving, drain sweet and sour juice from cucumber slices and place cucumbers into a serving bowl. 4 Servings.

PER SERVING – 1/2 CUP

Calories	44	Protein	0g
Total Fat	0g	Carbohydrate	11g
Saturated Fat	0g	Cholesterol	0mg
Sodium	268mg	Fiber	0g

EXCHANGES: 1 Starch

GREEN BEAN AND BABY CORN SALAD

1. **1 Pound Green Beans (trimmed)**
2. **1 Can (7 oz.) Picked Baby Ears of Corn (undrained)**
3. **4 Green Onion (sliced)**

Blanch beans for 5-6 minutes in salted water until crisp tender. Drain, rinse and cool. Combine with baby corn and onions. Juice from corn acts as dressing. Toss and chill. 6 Servings.

PER SERVING – 1/2 CUP

Calories	32	Protein	1g
Total Fat	0g	Carbohydrate	7g
Saturated Fat	0g	Cholesterol	0mg
Sodium	247mg	Fiber	2g

EXCHANGES: 1 1/2 Vegetable

SUNNY SPINACH SALAD

1. 1 Pound Spinach (torn into bite-size pieces)
2. 1 Medium Red Onion (thinly sliced)
3. 1 Package (6 oz.) Dried Apricots No Sugar (chopped)
4. 1/3 Cup Toasted Salted Sunflower Seeds

Combine ingredients. Good served with vinaigrette dressing. 6 Servings.

SERVING SIZE - 3/4 CUP

Calories	96	Protein	4g
Total Fat	5g	Carbohydrate	13g
Saturated Fat	0g	Cholesterol	0mg
Sodium	107mg	Fiber	5g

EXCHANGES: 1 Vegetable, 1/2 Fruit, 1 Fat

SPINACH SALAD

1. 1 Pound Spinach (torn in bite-size pieces)
2. 1 Medium Red Onion (thinly sliced)
3. 1 Can (11 oz.) Mandarin Oranges (drained)
4. 1/2 Cup Fat Free Wine Vinaigrette Salad Dressing

Combine ingredients. Refrigerate until ready to serve. 4 Servings.

PER SERVING – 1/2 CUP

Calories	87	Protein	5g
Total Fat	1g	Carbohydrate	17g
Saturated Fat	0g	Cholesterol	0mg
Sodium	473mg	Fiber	4g

EXCHANGES: 1 1/2 Vegetable, 1/2 Fruit

HEARTY SPINACH AND MUSHROOM SALAD

1. 1 Bag (10 oz.) Cold Water Washed Spinach (torn in bite-sized pieces)
2. 1 Package (8 oz.) Sliced Mushrooms
3. 1 Medium Zucchini (sliced)
4. 1/2 Cup Fat Free Red Wine Vinegar Dressing

In large bowl, toss spinach, mushrooms and zucchini. Add dressing and toss again. 8 Servings.

PER SERVING – 1/2 CUP

Calories	21	Protein	2g
Total Fat	0g	Carbohydrate	4g
Saturated Fat	0g	Cholesterol	0mg
Sodium	219mg	Fiber	1g

EXCHANGES: 1 Vegetable

SUNSHINE SALAD

1. 1 Package (10 oz.) Cold Water Washed Spinach (torn in bite-sized pieces)
2. 2 Navel Oranges (peeled, sectioned, cut in half)
3. 1/2 Red Onion (thinly sliced)
4. 1/2 Cup Sweet and Sour Dressing

Mix spinach, oranges and red onion. Toss with dressing and chill until ready to serve. 8 Servings.

PER SERVING – 3/4 CUP

Calories	57	Protein	2g
Total Fat	1g	Carbohydrate	13g
Saturated Fat	0g	Cholesterol	0mg
Sodium	97mg	Fiber	4g

EXCHANGES: 1 Vegetable, 1/2 Fruit

TANGY SPINACH SALAD

1. 1 Package (10 oz.) Cold Water Washed Spinach (torn in bite-sized pieces)
2. 1 Cup Fat Free Cottage Cheese
3. 1 Red Bell Pepper (thinly sliced)
4. 1/2 Cup Sweet and Sour Dressing

Combine above ingredients and toss with dressing. 8 Servings.

PER SERVING – 3/4 CUP

Calories	76	Protein	7g
Total Fat	1g	Carbohydrate	11g
Saturated Fat	0g	Cholesterol	6mg
Sodium	212mg	Fiber	1g

EXCHANGES: 1/2 Very Lean Meat, 2 Vegetable

SPINACH WITH SPROUTS

1. 1 Package (10 oz.) Cold Water Washed Spinach (torn in bite-sized pieces)
2. 2 Cups Fresh Bean Sprouts
3. 1 Can (8 1/2 oz.) Water Chestnuts (sliced, drained)
4. 1/2 Cup Fat Free Mayonnaise

Combine above ingredients and toss with mayonnaise. 8 Servings.

PER SERVING – 1/2 CUP

Calories	43	Protein	2g
Total Fat	0g	Carbohydrate	10g
Saturated Fat	0g	Cholesterol	0mg
Sodium	222mg	Fiber	1g

EXCHANGES: 1/2 Starch, 1 Vegetable

FRUIT AND SPINACH SALAD

1. 1 Package (10 oz.) Cold Water Washed Spinach
2. 1 Large Red Delicious Apple (cored, chopped)
3. 1 Medium Pear (cored, chopped)
4. 1/2 Cup Low Fat Honey Mustard Dressing

Combine above ingredients and toss with the low fat dressing. 8 Servings.

PER SERVING – 1/2 CUP

Calories	65	Protein	1g
Total Fat	1g	Carbohydrate	15g
Saturated Fat	0g	Cholesterol	0mg
Sodium	97mg	Fiber	2g

EXCHANGES: 1 Fruit, 1/2 Vegetable

ROMAINE STRAWBERRY SALAD

1. **4 Cups Romaine Lettuce (torn into bite-sized pieces)**
2. **1 Cup Fresh Strawberries (sliced)**
3. **1/2 Purple Onion (coarsely chopped)**
4. **1/4 Cup Fat Free Wine Vinaigrette Dressing**

Combine first three ingredients and toss gently. Serve with vinaigrette dressing. 6 Servings.

PER SERVING – 3/4 CUP

Calories	22	Protein	1g
Total Fat	0g	Carbohydrate	4g
Saturated Fat	0g	Cholesterol	0mg
Sodium	130mg	Fiber	1g

EXCHANGES: 1/3 Fruit

FROZEN PINEAPPLE CRANBERRY SALAD

1. 1 Can (20 oz.) Water Packed Crushed Pineapple (drained)
2. 1 Can (16 oz.) Whole Cranberry Sauce
3. 1 Cup Fat Free Sour Cream
4. 1/2 Cup Pecans (chopped)

Combine all ingredients and place in a 8x8-inch pan. Freeze, cut into squares before serving. 9 Servings.

SERVING SIZE - 1 SQUARE

Calories	150	Protein	4g
Total Fat	4g	Carbohydrate	27g
Saturated Fat	0g	Cholesterol	0m
Sodium	29mg	Fiber	2g

EXCHANGES: 1 1/2 Fruit, 1/2 Lean Meat, 1/2 Fat

PEA SALAD

1. **1 Package (10 oz.) Frozen Green Peas (thawed)**
2. **1/2 Cup Fat Free Cheddar Cheese (cubed)**
3. **1/2 Cup Celery (chopped)**
4. **1/2 Cup Fat Free Sour Cream**

Combine above ingredients. Salt and pepper to taste. Refrigerate for several hours. Serve on bed of lettuce. 6 Servings.

SERVING SIZE - 1/2 CUP

Calories	72	Protein	10g
Total Fat	0g	Carbohydrate	8g
Saturated Fat	0g	Cholesterol	3mg
Sodium	197mg	Fiber	2g

EXCHANGES: 1/2 Bread, 1 Very Lean Meat

WALDORF SALAD

1. **4 Cups Apples (chopped)**
2. **3/4 Cup Raisins**
3. **1/2 Cup Pecans (pieces)**
4. **1/2 Cup Lowfat Mayonnaise**

Combine ingredients. Refrigerate until ready to serve. 8 Servings.

SERVING SIZE - 3/4 CUP

Calories	187	Protein	1g
Total Fat	9g	Carbohydrate	29g
Saturated Fat	1g	Cholesterol	0mg
Sodium	115mg	Fiber	3g

EXCHANGES: 2 Breads, 2 Fats

APPLE SALAD WITH FETA CHEESE

1. 1 Large Head Bibb Lettuce (torn in bite-sized pieces)
2. 1 Large Red Delicious Apple (diced)
3. 2 Ounces Feta Cheese (crumbled)
4. 1/4 Cup Fat Free Wine Vinaigrette Dressing

Dice apples right before serving and toss with fat free Vinaigrette. Combine with other ingredients. 4 Servings.

PER SERVING – 1/2 CUP

Calories	93	Protein	3g
Total Fat	3g	Carbohydrate	12g
Saturated Fat	2g	Cholesterol	12mg
Sodium	362mg	Fiber	2g

EXCHANGES: 1/2 Vegetable, 1/2 Fruit, 1/2 Fat

LAYERED FRUIT SALAD

1. **3 Cups Orange Sections**
2. **1 Can (15 1/4 oz.) Crushed Pineapple (water packed)**
3. **1/2 Cup Flaked Coconut**
4. **1 Tablespoon Honey**

Drain pineapple. Layer 1 1/2 cups oranges, 1/2 pineapple, 1/4 cup coconut. Repeat layer. Drizzle with honey and cover. Chill overnight. 4 Servings.

PER SERVING – 1 CUP

Calories	159	Protein	2g
Total Fat	4g	Carbohydrate	31g
Saturated Fat	4g	Cholesterol	0mg
Sodium	33mg	Fiber	9g

EXCHANGES: 2 Fruit, 1 Fat

MANDARIN SALAD

1. 2 Tomatoes (peeled, sliced)
2. 2 Cans (11oz. each) Mandarin Oranges (drained)
3. 1/2 Cup Onion (thinly sliced)
4. 3 Cups Lettuce Leaves (torn into bite-size pieces)

Combine ingredients. Good served with Orange Juice Dressing. (Recipe follows.)

SERVING SIZE - 3/4 CUP

Calories	56	Protein	1g
Total Fat	0g	Carbohydrate	14g
Saturated Fat	0g	Cholesterol	0mg
Sodium	12mg	Fiber	1g

EXCHANGES: 1/2 Vegetable, 1/2 Fruit

ORANGE JUICE DRESSING

1. **1/4 Cup Orange Juice**
2. **2 Teaspoons Red Wine Vinegar**
3. **1 Tablespoon Canola Oil**
4. **2 Teaspoons Honey**

Mix above ingredients and pour over mandarin salad.

SERVING SIZE - 2 TABLESPOONS

Calories	33	Protein	0g
Total Fat	2g	Carbohydrate	3g
Saturated Fat	0g	Cholesterol	0mg
Sodium	1mg	Fiber	0g

EXCHANGES: 1/2 Fat

MUSHROOM SALAD

1. 1 Medium head Romaine Lettuce
2. 1 Cup Sliced Mushrooms
3. 1 Cup Cucumber (peeled and diced)
4. 1/4 Cup Fat Free Italian Salad Dressing

Tear the lettuce into bite-size pieces and place them in a salad bowl. Add the sliced mushrooms and cucumber. Toss with dressing. 6 Servings.

SERVING SIZE - 2 CUPS

Calories	48	Protein	4g
Total Fat	1g	Carbohydrate	8g
Saturated Fat	0g	Cholesterol	0mg
Sodium	159mg	Fiber	4g

EXCHANGES: 2 Vegetables

QUICK MELON SALAD

1. 1 Tablespoon Honey
2. 3 Tablespoons Lime Juice
3. 2 Cups Honeydew Melon (cubed or balls)
4. 2 Cups Cantaloupe (cubed or balls)

In a medium bowl, whisk together the honey and lime juice. Add all the melon and toss to coat thoroughly. Cover and refrigerate until very cold, about 1 hour. 4 Servings.

SERVING SIZE - 1 CUP

Calories	77	Protein	1g
Total Fat	0g	Carbohydrate	20g
Saturated Fat	0g	Cholesterol	0mg
Sodium	16mg	Fiber	1g

EXCHANGES: 1 Fruit

Vegetables

STUFFED BAKED POTATOES

1. **4 Baking Potatoes (baked)**
2. **1/2 Cup Skim Milk**
3. **2 Tablespoons Fat Free Margarine**
4. **1/4 Cup Fat Free Cheddar Cheese**

Cut baked potatoes in half lengthwise. Scoop potato out of skin leaving shell intact. Mash potato pulp with milk and margarine. Stir in cheese. Refill potato shells with mixture and reheat briefly at 350 degrees until warm. 8 Servings.

PER SERVING - 1/2 POTATO

Calories	127	Protein	5g
Total Fat	0g	Carbohydrate	27g
Saturated Fat	0g	Cholesterol	2mg
Sodium	89mg	Fiber	3g

EXCHANGES: 1 1/2 Starches, 1/2 Very Lean Meat

NEW POTATOES VINAIGRETTE

1. **2 Cans (16 oz.) New Potatoes**
2. **1/4 Cup Fat Free Vinaigrette Dressing**
3. **1 Tablespoon Fresh Parsley (chopped)**

Heat potatoes thoroughly. Drain. Place in bowl and toss gently with dressing. Sprinkle with parsley and serve. 6 Servings.

PER SERVING – 3/4 CUP

Calories	96	Protein	2g
Total Fat	0g	Carbohydrate	22g
Saturated Fat	0g	Cholesterol	0mg
Sodium	522mg	Fiber	4g

EXCHANGES: 1 1/2 Starches

HERBED NEW POTATOES

1. **2 Cans (15 oz.) New Potatoes**
2. **1 Tablespoon Minced Parsley**
3. **1 Tablespoon Minced Chives**
4. **1 Tablespoon Fat Free Margarine**

Heat potatoes in medium saucepan. Drain and add remaining ingredients, toss until potatoes are coated. 4 Servings.

PER SERVING – ONE CUP

Calories	132	Protein	3g
Total Fat	0g	Carbohydrate	30g
Saturated Fat	0g	Cholesterol	0mg
Sodium	580mg	Fiber	5g

EXCHANGES: 2 Starches

POTATOES O'BRIEN

1. **2 Cans (15 oz.) Sliced New Potatoes (drained)**
2. **1/2 Onion (finely minced)**
3. **1/2 Green Pepper (diced)**
4. **2 Tablespoons Fat Free Margarine**

Melt margarine in nonstick skillet. Add onions and green pepper and sauté over medium heat until tender. Add drained potatoes and continue to sauté for 5 minutes. Pepper to taste. 4 Servings.

PER SERVING – ONE CUP

Calories	145	Protein	3g
Total Fat	0g	Carbohydrate	33g
Saturated Fat	0g	Cholesterol	0mg
Sodium	599mg	Fiber	6g

EXCHANGES: 2 Starches, 1/2 Vegetable

ROASTED NEW POTATOES

1. 4 Medium Sized New Potatoes (quartered)
2. 2 Tablespoons Fat Free Margarine
3. 3 Small Onions (quartered)
4. 1/2 Teaspoon Marjoram

Melt margarine in an oven proof casserole. Stir in marjoram. Add potatoes and onions and toss in melted mixture until coated. Cover dish and bake at 400 degrees for 1 to 1 1/2 hours. 4 Servings.

PER SERVING – 1/2 CUP

Calories	108	Protein	3g
Total Fat	0g	Carbohydrate	24g
Saturated Fat	0g	Cholesterol	0mg
Sodium	55mg	Fiber	3g

EXCHANGES: 1 1/2 Starches, 1/2 Vegetable

SPICY NEW POTATOES

1. 8 Small New Potatoes
2. 1 Teaspoon Concentrated Instant Liquid Crab & Shrimp Boil
3. 4 Cups Water

Pour crab boil into water and bring to a boil. Puncture potatoes and add to boiling water. Reduce heat and simmer until potato skins barely pop and potatoes are tender, around 20 minutes. 6 Servings.

PER SERVING –1/2 CUP

Calories	77	Protein	3g
Total Fat	1g	Carbohydrate	16g
Saturated Fat	0g	Cholesterol	0mg
Sodium	248mg	Fiber	1g

EXCHANGES: 1 Starch

MASHED POTATOES AND CARROTS

1. 4 Potatoes (peeled, cut into chunks)
2. 1 Large Carrot (peeled, cut into chunks)
3. 1/3 Cup Skim Milk
4. 1 Teaspoon Dried Dill Leaves

In boiling water, add potatoes and carrot and cook for 25 minutes or until tender. Drain. Return to pot and mash. Stir in milk and dill. 6 Servings.

PER SERVING – 1/2 CUP

Calories	79	Protein	2g
Total Fat	0g	Carbohydrate	18g
Saturated Fat	0g	Cholesterol	0mg
Sodium	17mg	Fiber	1g

EXCHANGES: 1/2 Vegetable, 1 Starch

COTTAGE CHEESE STUFFED BAKED POTATOES

1. 2 Baking Potatoes (baked)
2. 1 Cup Lowfat Cottage Cheese
3. 1 Tablespoon Chives
4. 1 Teaspoon Onion Powder

Bake potatoes in 425 degrees oven for 1 hour. Cut potatoes in half lengthwise and scoop out insides. Return shell to oven and bake until crisp. Whip potato insides with remaining ingredients and put mixture into potato skins. Return to oven and bake until thoroughly heated. 4 Servings.

PER SERVING – 3/4 CUP

Calories	153	Protein	9g
Total Fat	1g	Carbohydrate	27g
Saturated Fat	0g	Cholesterol	3mg
Sodium	238mg	Fiber	3g

EXCHANGES: 1 Very Lean Meat, 1 1/2 Starches

COTTAGED SWEET POTATOES

1. **4 Sweet Potatoes (peeled, cut into strips)**
2. **2 Tablespoons Canola Oil**
3. **2 Tablespoons Cajun Spice Seasoning**
4. **1 Tablespoon Hot Pepper Sauce**

Mix oil, Cajun spice and hot pepper sauce together. Add potatoes and toss until well coated. Spread potatoes onto a nonstick pan sprayed lightly with cooking spray. Bake at 400 degrees for 40 minutes, turning occasionally, or until potatoes are tender. 8 Servings.

PER SERVING – 1/2 CUP

Calories	152	Protein	2g
Total Fat	4g	Carbohydrate	27g
Saturated Fat	0g	Cholesterol	0mg
Sodium	32mg	Fiber	0g

EXCHANGES: 1 1/2 Starches

GINGERED SWEET POTATOES

1. 2 Medium Sweet Potatoes (peeled, diced)
2. 1 Tablespoon Fat Free Margarine
3. 1 Teaspoon Brown Sugar
4. 1/4 Teaspoon Ground Ginger or Pumpkin Pie Spice

Arrange potatoes in a steaming rack. Place over boiling water; cover and steam until tender. Remove and place in serving dish. Combine remaining ingredients, blend well. Toss with the hot sweet potatoes. 4 Servings.

PER SERVING - 1/2 CUP

Calories	98	Protein	2g
Total Fat	0g	Carbohydrate	23g
Saturated Fat	0g	Cholesterol	0mg
Sodium	32mg	Fiber	3g

EXCHANGES: 1 1/2 Starches

SCALLOPED POTATOES

1. **3 Medium Potatoes (thinly sliced)**
2. **1/3 Cup Grated Parmesan Cheese**
3. **2/3 Cup Skim Milk**
4. **1/2 Teaspoon Paprika**

Layer potatoes and cheese in a 2 quart casserole sprayed with nonstick spray. Pour milk over potatoes and sprinkle with paprika. Cover and vent. Cook in microwave for 12 minutes. Take out, remove cover and broil 2-3 minutes to brown. 4 Servings.

PER SERVING - 1/2 CUP

Calories	217	Protein	8g
Total Fat	3g	Carbohydrate	41g
Saturated Fat	2g	Cholesterol	7mg
Sodium	186mg	Fiber	4g

EXCHANGES: 2 Starches, 1/2 Lean Meat

CHILI BAKED FRIES

1. **4 Large Potatoes**
2. **2 Teaspoons Butter Buds (made into liquid)**
3. **2 Teaspoons Chili Powder**

Cut potatoes into strips. Arrange on a baking sheet that has been sprayed with nonstick spray. Dip each strip into liquid butter buds or brush with butter buds mixture on potato. Sprinkle chili powder on top. Bake at 425 degrees for 15-20 minutes or until golden brown. Turn, bake another 15-20 minutes or until tender. 4 Servings.

SERVING SIZE - 1 CUP

Calories	73	Protein	1g
Total Fat	0g	Carbohydrate	16g
Saturated Fat	0g	Cholesterol	0mg
Sodium	197mg	Fiber	3g

EXCHANGES: 1 Starch

ITALIAN EGGPLANT

1. 1 Small Eggplant
2. 1/4 Cup Liquid Egg Substitute
3. 1/2 Cup Italian Seasoned Breadcrumbs
4. 1 1/2 Cup Spaghetti Sauce

Spray skillet with nonstick spray. Remove peel of eggplant and slice into circles. Dip circle in egg beater then into breadcrumbs. Place each round in skillet and brown on both sides. Place in ovenproof casserole, putting a generous tablespoon of spaghetti sauce on each eggplant round. Stack if necessary. Bake covered at 350 degrees for 30 minutes.
4 Servings.

PER SERVING - 1/2 CUP (1 CIRCLE)

Calories	142	Protein	5g
Total Fat	5g	Carbohydrate	20g
Saturated Fat	1g	Cholesterol	0mg
Sodium	883mg	Fiber	2g

EXCHANGES: 1 1/2 Starches, 1/2 Fat

GARLIC GREEN BEANS

1. 1 Package (10 oz.) Frozen Italian-style Green Beans
2. 2 Teaspoons Olive Oil
3. 2 Garlic Cloves (crushed)
4. 2 Tablespoons Grated Parmesan Cheese

In nonstick skillet over medium heat, combine beans, olive oil and garlic. Bring to a boil. Cover, reduce heat and simmer 5 minutes. Remove cover, stir and cook 3 minutes longer or until liquid evaporates. Season to taste and sprinkle with Parmesan cheese. 4 Servings.

PER SERVING - 1/2 CUP

Calories	55	Protein	2g
Total Fat	3g	Carbohydrate	5g
Saturated Fat	1g	Cholesterol	2mg
Sodium	68mg	Fiber	2g

EXCHANGES: 1 Vegetable, 1/2 Fat (mono unsaturated)

GREEN BEANS WITH DILL

1. 2 Cans (14 1/2 oz.) French Style Green Beans
2. 1/2 cup Fresh Mushrooms (sliced)
3. 1 Teaspoon Fat Free Margarine
4. 1 1/2 Teaspoon Dried Dill Weed

Warm beans over medium to low heat. Add mushrooms and cook 1 minute longer. Drain and toss with margarine and dill. 6 Servings.

PER SERVING – 1/2 CUP

Calories	17	Protein	1g
Total Fat	0g	Carbohydrate	4g
Saturated Fat	0g	Cholesterol	0mg
Sodium	188mg	Fiber	2g

EXCHANGES: 1 Vegetable

CANDIED ACORN SQUASH

1. 2 Acorn Squash
2. 4 Tablespoons Lite Maple Syrup
3. 2 Teaspoons Fat Free Margarine
4. 1/4 Teaspoon Ground Allspice

Cut squash in half and remove seeds and stringy parts. Place halves, cut side up, in baking dish. Put 1 teaspoon syrup and 1/2 teaspoon margarine in each half. Sprinkle with allspice, cover and bake at 375 degrees for 35 minutes. 8 Servings.

PER SERVING - 1/4 OF SQUASH

Calories	42	Protein	1g
Total Fat	0g	Carbohydrate	11g
Saturated Fat	0g	Cholesterol	0mg
Sodium	39mg	Fiber	1g

EXCHANGES: 1/2 Starches

SKILLET SQUASH

1. **1 Medium Acorn Squash**
2. **1/3 Cup Pineapple Juice**
3. **1 Tablespoon Brown Sugar**
4. **1/4 Teaspoon Cinnamon**

Cut squash crosswise into 1/2-inch slices and discard seeds. Arrange in large skillet. In small bowl, combine juice, sugar and cinnamon. Pour over squash rings. Bring to a boil and reduce heat. Simmer, covered, for 25 minutes or until squash is tender. Arrange squash on platter and pour remaining sauce over squash. 4 Servings.

PER SERVING – 1/2 CUP

Calories	82	Protein	1g
Total Fat	0g	Carbohydrate	21g
Saturated Fat	0g	Cholesterol	0mg
Sodium	6mg	Fiber	2g

EXCHANGES: 1 1/2 Starches

ZUCCHINI SQUASH

1. **2 Medium Zucchini Squash**
2. **Butter Flavored Spray**
3. **4 Teaspoons Parmesan Cheese**
4. **4 Teaspoons Seasoned Bread Crumbs**

Place zucchini on microwaveable dish. Pierce with fork. Microwave approximately 5 minutes on high temperature or until tender, but not soft. Split in half lengthwise. Spray with butter spray. Sprinkle each half with 1 teaspoon cheese and 1 teaspoon bread crumbs. 4 Servings.

PER SERVING – 1/2 CUP

Calories	36	Protein	2g
Total Fat	1g	Carbohydrate	5g
Saturated Fat	0g	Cholesterol	2mg
Sodium	62mg	Fiber	1g

EXCHANGES: 1 Vegetable

SESAME RICE

1. 4 Cups White Rice (cooked)
2. 1/4 Cup Green Onions (chopped)
3. 2 Tablespoon Sesame Seeds
4. 1/4 Cup Low Sodium Soy Sauce

While rice is still hot, combine all ingredients and place into serving dish. Stir well. 8 Servings.

PER SERVING - 1/2 CUP

Calories	100	Protein	3g
Total Fat	1g	Carbohydrate	19g
Saturated Fat	0g	Cholesterol	0mg
Sodium	303mg	Fiber	1g

EXCHANGES: 1 Starch, 1/2 Fat (mono unsaturated)

SPINACH CASSEROLE

1. 1 Carton (16 oz.) Fat Free Cottage Cheese
2. 8 Ounces Fat Free Cheddar Cheese (grated)
3. 1 Package (10 oz.) Chopped Spinach (drained)
4. 3/4 Cup Egg Substitute

Combine all ingredients and mix well. Spoon into casserole sprayed with nonstick spray. Bake 45 minutes at 350 degrees. 6 Servings.

PER SERVING - 1 CUP

Calories	127	Protein	25g
Total Fat	0g	Carbohydrate	7g
Saturated Fat	0g	Cholesterol	10 mg
Sodium	633 mg	Fiber	1g

EXCHANGES: 1/2 Vegetables, 3 1/2 Very Lean Meats

SAUTEED SPINACH

1. 1 Pound Fresh Spinach
2. 1 Tablespoons Olive Oil
3. 2 Tablespoons White Wine or Cooking Sherry
4. 1/4 Cup Freshly Grated Parmesan Cheese

Wash and dry spinach. Cook spinach in olive oil in large skillet over high heat. Stir constantly until wilted. Add wine and cook until liquid is gone. Sprinkle with Parmesan cheese and serve.
4 Servings.

PER SERVING - 1/2 CUP

Calorie	121	Protein	8g
Total Fat	7g	Carbohydrate	5g
Saturated Fat	1g	Cholesterol	9mg
Sodium	316mg	Fiber	3g

EXCHANGES: 1 Vegetable, 1 Fat

SPINACH TOPPED TOMATOES

1. 1 Package (10 oz.) Chopped Spinach (cooked, drained)
2. 1 Teaspoon Low Salt Instant Chicken Bouillon
3. 1/4 Teaspoon Nutmeg
4. 3 Medium Tomatoes

Place spinach in medium bowl. Mix bouillon with 1/2 cup hot water. Combine spinach with broth and nutmeg. Cut tomatoes into halves crosswise and arrange, cut side up, on baking sheet. Top each tomato half with 1/6 of the spinach mixture. Bake at 325 degrees for 30 minutes or until tomatoes are tender, but retain their shape. 6 Servings.

PER SERVING – ONE CUP

Calories	34	Protein	3g
Total Fat	0g	Carbohydrate	6g
Saturated Fat	0g	Cholesterol	0mg
Sodium	60mg	Fiber	1g

EXCHANGES: 1 Vegetable

TOMATO STACK

1 1 Package (10 oz.) Frozen Chopped Broccoli
2. 1 Cup Lowfat Grated Monterrey Jack Cheese
3. 1/4 Cup Onion (finely chopped)
4. 3 Large Tomatoes (halved)

Cook broccoli as directed. Drain and mix with cheese, reserve 2 tablespoons of cheese for top. Add onion. Place tomato halves in greased baking dish. Place broccoli mixture on each tomato half and top with reserved cheese. Broil 10-12 minutes at 350 degrees. 6 Servings.

PER SERVING - 1/2 TOMATO

Calories	135	Protein	13g
Total Fat	8g	Carbohydrate	6g
Saturated Fat	4g	Cholesterol	27mg
Sodium	144mg	Fiber	3g

EXCHANGES: 1 Vegetable, 1 1/2 Lean Meat, 1/2 Fat

HERB TOMATO SLICES

1. **3 Medium Tomatoes**
2. **2/3 Cups Fresh Bread Crumbs**
3. **1 Tablespoon Fat Free Margarine (melted)**
4. **1/4 Teaspoon Dried Basil**

Slice tomatoes and place in shallow baking dish. Mix bread crumbs, margarine and basil. Sprinkle mixture over tomatoes and bake, uncovered, at 350 degrees for 5-6 minutes or until crumbs are brown.
6 Servings.

PER SERVING – 1/2 CUP

Calories	33	Protein	2g
Total Fat	0g	Carbohydrate	6g
Saturated Fat	0g	Cholesterol	0mg
Sodium	54mg	Fiber	1g

EXCHANGES: 1/2 Vegetable, 1/2 Starch

COLD VEGETABLE DISH

1. 1 Basket Cherry Tomatoes
2. 1 Bunch Broccoli (fresh and cut up)
3. 1 Head Cauliflower (fresh and cut up)
4. 1 Bottle (8 oz.) Fat Free Italian Salad Dressing

Mix above ingredients the day before you are ready to serve. Serve cold. 8 Servings.

PER SERVING – 1/2 CUP

Calories	36	Protein	2g
Total Fat	0g	Carbohydrate	7g
Saturated Fat	0g	Cholesterol	0mg
Sodium	415mg	Fiber	1g

EXCHANGES: 1 1/2 Vegetables

MARINATED VEGETABLES

1. 1 Package (10 oz.) Frozen Cut Green Beans
2. 1 Package (10 oz.) Frozen Cauliflower
3. 1/4 Cup Fat Free Italian Dressing
4. 1 Jar (2 oz.) Sliced Pimiento (drained)

Cook beans and cauliflower according to package directions. Drain vegetables and place in mixing bowl. Add salad dressing and pimiento. Toss until vegetables are coated. Cover and chill at least 4 hours or overnight. 8 Servings.

PER SERVING – ONE CUP

Calories	41	Protein	2g
Total Fat	0g	Carbohydrate	9g
Saturated Fat	0g	Cholesterol	0mg
Sodium	126mg	Fiber	1g

EXCHANGES: 2 Vegetables

BAKED ONION RINGS

1. **1/2 Cup Liquid Egg Substitute**
2. **1 Large Sweet Yellow Onion (cut into rings)**
3. **1/3 Cup Dry Bread Crumbs (plain or seasoned)**
4. **Salt And Pepper To Taste**

Mix egg substitute, salt and pepper. Dip onion rings into egg mixture and then coat with breadcrumbs. Place in single layer on greased baking sheet. Bake 10 minutes at 450 degrees. 4 Servings.

PER SERVING - 1/2 CUP

Calories	72	Protein	3g
Total Fat	1g	Carbohydrate	14g
Saturated Fat	0g	Cholesterol	0mg
Sodium	100 mg	Fiber	1g

EXCHANGES: 1 Vegetable, 1/2 Starch

SAUTEED BROCCOLI

1. 1 Package (10 oz.) Frozen Broccoli
2. 1 Package (10 oz.) Frozen Whole Kernel Corn
3. 1 Can (4 oz.) Sliced Mushrooms (drained)
4. 2 Tablespoons Fat Free Margarine

Melt margarine in large nonstick skillet. Sauté broccoli, corn and mushrooms in melted margarine until crisp-tender. Serve warm. Season to taste.
4 Servings.

PER SERVING – 1/2 CUP

Calories	84	Protein	5g
Total Fat	0g	Carbohydrate	20g
Saturated Fat	0g	Cholesterol	0mg
Sodium	184mg	Fiber	4g

EXCHANGES: 1 Vegetable, 1 Starch

ITALIAN STYLE BROCCOLI

1. 1 1/2 Pounds Broccoli (cut into flowerets)
2. Olive Oil Fat Free Cooking Spray
3. 2 Cloves Garlic (minced)
4. 2 Tablespoons Lemon Juice

Steam broccoli in large skillet for 5 minutes until crisp-tender. Remove broccoli and drain. Spray skillet with cooking spray and add garlic. Cook over medium heat stirring constantly until garlic is lightly browned. Add broccoli and lemon juice. Toss gently. Cover and cook for an additional minute. 4 Servings.

PER SERVING – ONE CUP

Calories	53	Protein	5g
Total Fat	1g	Carbohydrate	10g
Saturated Fat	0g	Cholesterol	0mg
Sodium	48mg	Fiber	6g

EXCHANGES: 2 Vegetables

DIJON BROCCOLI

1. **1 Cup Uncooked Pasta (about 4 ounces)**
2. **1 Package (10 oz.) Frozen Chopped Broccoli (cooked and drained)**
3. **1/4 Cup Fat Free Sour Cream**
4. **2 Tablespoons Dijon Mustard**

Cook pasta according to package directions. Drain. Combine broccoli, sour cream and mustard with pasta. Toss all ingredients until well mixed. Chill until ready to serve. 6 Servings.

PER SERVING – 1/2 CUP

Calories	131	Protein	7g
Total Fat	3g	Carbohydrate	18g
Saturated Fat	0g	Cholesterol	18mg
Sodium	864mg	Fiber	2g

EXCHANGES: 1/2 Vegetable, 1 Starch

PARMESAN BROCCOLI AND MUSHROOMS

1. 1 Package (10 oz.) Frozen Chopped Broccoli (cooked and drained)
2. 1 Jar (4 1/2 oz.) Sliced Mushrooms (drained)
3. 2 Tablespoons Fat Free Margarine
4. 1/4 Cup Grated Parmesan Cheese

While broccoli is still warm, combine above ingredients. Toss and serve. 4 Servings.

PER SERVING – 1/2 CUP

Calories	56	Protein	5g
Total Fat	2g	Carbohydrate	6g
Saturated Fat	1g	Cholesterol	5mg
Sodium	312mg	Fiber	3g

EXCHANGES: 1 Vegetable, 1/2 Lean Meat

CHEESY CAULIFLOWER

1. 1 Bag (16 oz.) Frozen Cauliflower (cooked, drained)
2. 1/2 Cup Cream of Chicken Soup - Condensed
3. 1/4 Cup Skim Milk
4. 1 Cup Low Fat, Low Sodium, Swiss Cheese (shredded)

Place cauliflower in baking dish. Combine soup, milk and cheese and spread over cauliflower. Bake for 10 minutes at 350 degrees. 4 Servings.

PER SERVING - 1/2 CUP

Calorie	218	Protein	21g
Total Fat	8g	Carbohydrate	9g
Saturated Fat	5g	Cholesterol	23mg
Sodium	375mg	Fiber	2g

EXCHANGES: 1 Vegetable, 2 1/2 Lean Meats, 1/2 Fats

LEMON BRUSSELS SPROUTS

1. 1 Package (10 oz.) Frozen Brussels Sprouts
2. 2 Teaspoons Fat Free Margarine
3. 2 Teaspoons Chopped Parsley
4. 2 Teaspoons Grated Lemon Rind

Prepare brussels sprouts according to package directions. Drain and place in serving bowl. In small saucepan, melt margarine and stir in parsley and lemon rind. Heat and pour over sprouts. 4 Servings.

PER SERVING – 1/2 CUP

Calories	41	Protein	3g
Total Fat	0g	Carbohydrate	8g
Saturated Fat	0g	Cholesterol	0mg
Sodium	116mg	Fiber	3g

EXCHANGES: 1 1/2 Vegetables

HOT CABBAGE

1. 3 Cups Cabbage (finely chopped)
2. 1/2 Teaspoon Salt
3. 2 Tablespoons Canola Oil
4. 2 Tablespoons Fat Free Italian Salad Dressing

Sprinkle cabbage with salt and set aside for 30 minutes. Heat oil in skillet until very hot. Add the cabbage and stir fry about 2 minutes. Remove and add Italian dressing. 4 Servings.

PER SERVING – 1/2 – 3/4 CUP

Calories	77	Protein	1g
Total Fat	7g	Carbohydrate	4g
Saturated Fat	0g	Cholesterol	0mg
Sodium	406mg	Fiber	1g

EXCHANGES: 1 Vegetable, 1 1/2 Fats

OKRA SUCCOTASH

1. **3 Cups Okra (sliced)**
2. **1 Can (16 oz.) Corn**
3. **1 Can (14 1/2 oz.) Seasoned Stewed Tomatoes**
4. **1/2 Cup Onion (chopped)**

Rinse okra under running water. Drain. Combine ingredients in a large skillet. Cover and simmer for 15 minutes. Season to taste. 6 Servings.

PER SERVING – ONE CUP

Calories	110	Protein	4g
Total Fat	1g	Carbohydrate	25g
Saturated Fat	0g	Cholesterol	0mg
Sodium	423mg	Fiber	3g

EXCHANGES: 2 Vegetables, 1 Starch

ASPARAGUS IN LEMON BUTTER

1. **1 Pound Asparagus (remove tough stems)**
2. **2 Tablespoons Fat Free Margarine (melted)**
3. **1/2 Teaspoon Fresh Grated Lemon Peel**
4. **2 Tablespoons Fresh Lemon Juice**

Cut asparagus in pieces about 1 1/2-inches long. Simmer asparagus in water, enough to cover, for about 6 minutes or until crisp tender. Drain. In saucepan combine all ingredients. Cook over medium heat for 2 minutes. Stir and serve warm. 4 Servings.

PER SERVING - 1/2 CUP

Calorie	31	Protein	3g
Total Fat	0g	Carbohydrate	6g
Saturated Fat	0g	Cholesterol	0mg
Sodium	51mg	Fiber	0g

EXCHANGES: 1 Vegetable

LEMON ASPARAGUS AND BABY CARROTS

1. 1 Pound Asparagus (steamed until crisp tender)
2. 1/2 Pound Small Carrots (steamed until crisp tender)
3. Lemon Pepper
4. 1 Tablespoon Lemon Juice

Drain asparagus and carrots. In casserole, combine carrots and asparagus. Cover and refrigerate. When ready to serve, sprinkle with lemon pepper and lemon juice. Serve cold. 4 Servings.

PER SERVING – ONE CUP

Calories	53	Protein	4g
Total Fat	0g	Carbohydrate	11g
Saturated Fat	0g	Cholesterol	0mg
Sodium	33mg	Fiber	1g

EXCHANGES: 2 Vegetables

TARRAGON ASPARAGUS

1. **1 Pound Fresh Asparagus Spears**
2. **I Can't Believe It's Not Butter Spray**
3. **1 Tablespoon Tarragon**
4. **1/4 Teaspoon Pepper**

Wash asparagus and break off at tender point. Steam over boiling water for 6 minutes or until barely tender. Remove from heat and drain. Spray with butter spray and sprinkle with tarragon and pepper. 4 Servings.

PER SERVING – 1/2 CUP

Calories	34	Protein	3g
Total Fat	1g	Carbohydrate	5g
Saturated Fat	0g	Cholesterol	0mg
Sodium	13mg	Fiber	0g

EXCHANGES: 1 Vegetable

ASPARAGUS WITH SESAME SEEDS

1. 1 Pound Fresh Asparagus Spears
2. 2 Tablespoons Lime Juice
3. 1 Tablespoon Sesame Seeds
4. Pimiento Strips

Wash asparagus and break off at tender point. In large saucepan bring 1/2 cup water to a boil and add asparagus. Cover and steam until just tender, around 6 minutes. Remove from heat and drain. Place on platter, decorate with pimiento strips and sprinkle with lime juice and sesame seeds. Serve warm or cold. 4 Servings.

PER SERVING – 1/2 CUP

Calories	90	Protein	5g
Total Fat	4g	Carbohydrate	12g
Saturated Fat	1g	Cholesterol	0mg
Sodium	25mg	Fiber	2g

EXCHANGES: 1 Vegetable, 1/2 Starch, 1/2 Very Lean Meat, 1 Fat

FRENCH ONION RICE

1. 1 Cup Long Grain White Rice
2. 1/4 Cup Fat Free Margarine
3. 1 Can Onion Soup plus 1 Can Water
4. 1 Can (4 oz.) Chopped Mushrooms

Lightly brown rice in margarine. Add soup, water and mushrooms. Cover and simmer about 25 minutes or until liquid is gone. Fluff and serve. For less sodium, use fresh mushrooms instead of canned. 6 Servings.

PER SERVING - 1/2 CUP

Calorie	133	Protein	3g
Total Fat	1g	Carbohydrate	28g
Saturated Fat	0g	Cholesterol	0mg
Sodium	365mg	Fiber	1g

EXCHANGES: 2 Starches

CORN RELISH

LOW CARB

1. **2 Cans (11 oz. each) Mexican-style Corn**
2. **Sugar Substitute**
3. **1/3 Cup Cider Vinegar**
4. **1/3 Cup Sweet Pickle Relish**

Combine above ingredients and bring to a boil. Simmer for 5 minutes. Remove from heat, cover and refrigerate. 5 Servings.

PER SERVING - 1/2 CUP

Calories	130	Protein	3g
Total Fat	1g	Carbohydrate	31g
Saturated Fat	0g	Cholesterol	0mg
Sodium	532mg	Fiber	2g

EXCHANGES: 2 Starches

SOUTHWESTERN CORN

1. **2 Cans (15.25 oz.) Corn (drained)**
2. **1 Red Bell Pepper (chopped)**
3. **1/4 Cup Onions (chopped)**
4. **Butter Flavored Spray**

Spray nonstick skillet with butter spray. Sauté pepper and onions in butter spray until soft. Add corn and cook over low heat for 10 minutes.
6 Servings.

PER SERVING – 1/2 CUP

Calories	128	Protein	4g
Total Fat	2g	Carbohydrate	15g
Saturated Fat	0g	Cholesterol	0mg
Sodium	466mg	Fiber	3g

EXCHANGES: 2 Starches

SPICY CORN BAKE

1. 2 Cans (15.25 oz.) Corn (drained)
2. 1/2 Cup Onion (sliced)
3. 1 Tablespoon Prepared Mustard
4. 1/2 Cup Chili Sauce

Sauté onion in nonstick skillet. Combine with remaining ingredients and place into a casserole. Bake at 350 degrees for 25 minutes. 6 Servings.

PER SERVING – 1/2 CUP

Calories	146	Protein	5g
Total Fat	2g	Carbohydrate	33g
Saturated Fat	0g	Cholesterol	0mg
Sodium	766mg	Fiber	3g

EXCHANGES: 2 Starches

MARVELOUS MUSHROOMS

1. **1 Pound Fresh Mushrooms (remove stems)**
2. **2 Tablespoons Canola Oil**
3. **2 1/2 Tablespoons Chopped Garlic**
4. **2 Tablespoons Lite Soy Sauce**

Cut mushroom stems off. Heat oil in frying pan and add garlic. Cook garlic over medium-low heat around 4-6 minutes. Do not let garlic burn. Add mushrooms and cook 2-3 minutes. Add soy sauce; toss and serve immediately. 4 Servings.

PER SERVING - 1/2 CUP

Calories	95	Protein	3g
Total Fat	7g	Carbohydrate	7g
Saturated Fat	1g	Cholesterol	0mg
Sodium	317mg	Fiber	2g

EXCHANGES: 1 1/2 Vegetables, 1 1/2 Fat

TANGY ITALIAN MUSHROOMS

1. 2 Cups Fresh Mushrooms (sliced)
2. 1/2 Cup Fat Free Italian Dressing
3. 1 Large Onion (chopped)
4. Butter Spray

Marinate mushrooms in dressing for at least 1 hour or overnight, stirring occasionally. In nonstick skillet, sauté onion in butter spray. Drain mushrooms and add to onions. Continue to cook over medium heat until mushrooms are tender, but not limp.
6 Servings.

PER SERVING – 1/2 CUP

Calories	25	Protein	1g
Total Fat	0g	Carbohydrate	5g
Saturated Fat	0g	Cholesterol	0mg
Sodium	282mg	Fiber	1g

EXCHANGES: 1 Vegetable

SESAME SNOW PEAS

1. **1 Pound Snow Pea Pods**
2. **1 Large Raw Carrot (scraped)**
3. **1 Teaspoon Vegetable Oil**
4. **1/2 Teaspoon Freshly Grated Orange Rind**

Place pea pods and carrots in a strainer. Set the strainer in a sink. Run very hot or boiling water over vegetables for about 1 minute, then pat dry. Place vegetables in a medium-sized bowl and stir in orange rind and oil. Serve warm or at room temperature. 4 Servings.

SERVING SIZE - 1/2 CUP

Calories	53	Protein	3g
Total Fat	1g	Carbohydrate	8g
Saturated Fat	0g	Cholesterol	0g
Sodium	10mg	Fiber	3g

EXCHANGES: 1/2 Vegetable, 1/2 Starch

SNOW PEAS AND MUSHROOMS

1. **1 Cup Sliced Mushrooms**
2. **2 Tablespoons Fat Free Margarine**
3. **1/2 Pound Small Snow Peas**
4. **1 Tablespoon Soy Sauce**

Sauté mushrooms in margarine. Stir in snow peas and soy sauce. Cook until crisp-tender. Toss and serve. 4 Servings.

PER SERVING – 1/2 CUP

Calories	37	Protein	5g
Total Fat	0g	Carbohydrate	4g
Saturated Fat	0g	Cholesterol	0mg
Sodium	367mg	Fiber	1g

EXCHANGES: 1 Vegetable

GINGER CARROTS

1. **1 Pound Carrots**
2. **1 Tablespoon Fat Free Margarine**
3. **1 Packet Equal**
4. **1 Teaspoon Grated Ginger**

Rinse, trim and peel carrots. Cut into 1/4-inch slices. Steam 15-20 minutes, or until barely tender. In a skillet over medium heat, melt margarine until it bubbles. Add drained carrots and toss. Sprinkle with sugar substitute and ginger. Toss again to coat carrots lightly. Continue to cook in skillet for another 1-2 minutes, or until carrots are lightly glazed.
5 Servings.

SERVING SIZE - 1/2 CUP

Calories	42	Protein	1g
Total Fat	0g	Carbohydrate	10g
Saturated Fat	0g	Cholesterol	0mg
Sodium	50mg	Fiber	2g

EXCHANGES: 2 Vegetables

PEACHY CARROTS

1. **1 Pound Package Carrots (sliced and cooked)**
2. **1/3 Cup Peach Preserves**
3. **1 Tablespoon Fat Free Margarine (melted)**

Combine carrots with margarine and peach preserves. Cook over low heat until carrots are heated thoroughly. 6 Servings.

PER SERVING – 3/4 CUP

Calories	38	Protein	1g
Total Fat	0g	Carbohydrate	9g
Saturated Fat	0g	Cholesterol	0mg
Sodium	42mg	Fiber	2g

EXCHANGES: 1 1/2 Vegetables

CARROT CASSEROLE I

1. **1 Pound Package Carrots (sliced, cooked tender)**
2. **1/2 Cup Celery (chopped)**
3. **1/3 Cup Onion (chopped)**
4. **1/3 Cup Green Pepper (chopped)**

Sauté chopped celery, onion and green pepper until tender. Mash cooked carrots and mix with sautéed vegetables. Put in baking dish sprayed with fat free cooking spray. Bake 30 minutes at 350 degrees. 6 Servings.

PER SERVING – ONE CUP

Calories	42	Protein	1g
Total Fat	0g	Carbohydrate	10g
Saturated Fat	0g	Cholesterol	0mg
Sodium	42mg	Fiber	2g

EXCHANGES: 2 Vegetables

CARROT CASSEROLE II

1. 1 Package (1 lb.) Mini Carrots (sliced)
2. 1/2 Cup Lowfat, Low Sodium Swiss Cheese (shredded)
3. 1/4 Teaspoon Ground Nutmeg
4. 1 Cup Low Sodium Chicken Broth

Cook carrots in broth until tender. Drain and retain broth. Mash carrots. Combine mashed carrots, cheese and nutmeg. Add 1/2 cup broth to make carrots creamy. Place in casserole and bake at 350 degrees for 15-20 minutes. 4 Servings.

PER SERVING – 1/2 CUP

Calories	145	Protein	12g
Total Fat	5g	Carbohydrate	12g
Saturated Fat	3g	Cholesterol	20mg
Sodium	116mg	Fiber	3g

EXCHANGES: 2 Vegetables, 1 1/2 Lean Meats

MINTED CARROTS

1. **3 Cups Sliced Carrots (cooked until crisp-tender)**
2. **1 Tablespoon Honey**
3. **1 Teaspoon Fresh or Dried Mint Leaves**
4. **Butter Flavored Spray**

Drain carrots and toss with honey, mint and butter spray. 6 Servings.

PER SERVING – 1/2 CUP

Calories	59	Protein	1g
Total Fat	0g	Carbohydrate	14g
Saturated Fat	0g	Cholesterol	0mg
Sodium	38mg	Fiber	3g

EXCHANGES: 2 1/2 Vegetables

CARROTS AND ZUCCHINI

1. 3 Medium Carrots (peeled and sliced)
2. 1 Medium Zucchini (sliced)
3. 1/2 Cup Low Sodium Chicken Broth
4. 1 Teaspoon Italian Seasoning

In saucepan cook carrots and zucchini in chicken broth until just tender. Drain. Add seasoning and toss gently. 4 Servings.

PER SERVING – 1/2 CUP

Calories	31	Protein	1g
Total Fat	0g	Carbohydrate	7g
Saturated Fat	0g	Cholesterol	1mg
Sodium	99mg	Fiber	2g

EXCHANGES: 1 1/2 Vegetables

BRAISED CELERY

1. **2 Cups Celery Sticks**
2. **1/2 Cup Beef Bouillon**
3. **2 Tablespoons Chopped Fresh Parsley**
4. **1 Tablespoon Fat Free Margarine**

Combine above ingredients and place in 1 quart casserole. Cover and bake at 400 degrees for 30 minutes. 4 Servings.

PER SERVING – 1/2 CUP

Calories	26	Protein	2g
Total Fat	0g	Carbohydrate	5g
Saturated Fat	0g	Cholesterol	0mg
Sodium	221mg	Fiber	2g

EXCHANGES: 1 Vegetable

Chicken

YOGURT CUMIN CHICKEN

1. **4 (3 oz.) Chicken Breasts (boneless, skinless)**
2. **1/3 Cup Nonfat Yogurt**
3. **1/4 Cup Sugar Free Apricot Jelly**
4. **1 Teaspoon Cumin**

Place chicken in baking dish that has been sprayed with nonstick spray. Bake, uncovered, for 30 minutes at 350 degrees. Mix yogurt, apricot jelly and cumin. Spoon over chicken. Bake for 15 minute or until chicken is no longer pink and sauce is heated.
4 Servings.

SERVING SIZE - ONE

Calories	149	Protein	27g
Total Fat	3g	Carbohydrate	1g
Saturated Fat	1g	Cholesterol	73m
Sodium	66mg	Fiber	0g

EXCHANGES: 3 Very Lean Meat

TARRAGON CHICKEN

1. 6 (5 oz.) Chicken Breasts (boneless, skinless)
2. 1 Cup White Cooking Wine
3. 1 Tablespoon Dried Tarragon Leaves
4. 2 Teaspoons Garlic Power

Combine wine, tarragon and garlic powder. Pour over chicken and marinate for several hours in refrigerator. Bake chicken at 350 degrees for 1 hour. 6 Servings.

SERVING SIZE - ONE

Calories	269	Protein	45g
Total Fat	5g	Carbohdrate	1g
Saturated Fat	1g	Cholesterol	122mg
Sodium	108mg	Fiber	0

EXCHANGES: 6 Very Lean Meat

BAKED CHIMICHANGAS

1. 8 (6 inch) Fat Free Flour Tortillas
2. 1 1/2 Cups Cooked and Cubed Chicken
3. 2 Ounces Grated Low Fat Cheese
4. 3/4 Cup Thick and Chunky Salsa

Mix chicken, cheese and salsa. Warm tortillas until pliable in 400 degree oven or 5 seconds each in microwave. Dampen one side of tortilla with water and place wet side down. Spoon on chicken mixture. Fold to hold in filling. Spray baking dish with nonstick spray. Lay chimichangas, seam side down, on baking dish. Bake for 15 minutes. 4 Servings.

SERVING SIZE - ONE

Calories	296	Protein	25g
Total Fat	4g	Carbohydrate	41g
Saturated Fat	2g	Cholesterol	43mg
Sodium	726mg	Fiber	1g

EXCHANGES: 2 1/2 Starches, 2 1/2 Very Lean Meat

ORANGE CHICKEN

1. 4 (6 oz.) Chicken Breasts (boneless, skinless)
2. 1 Cup Sugar Free Orange Soda
3. 1/4 Cup Low Sodium Soy Sauce
4. 4 Green Onions (finely chopped)

Combine soda and soy sauce. Marinate chicken breasts in mixture at least 8 hours or overnight in refrigerator. Place chicken and marinade in large baking dish. Sprinkle with onions and bake at 350 degrees for 1 hour. Baste occasionally. 4 Servings.

SERVING SIZE - ONE

Calorie	272	Protein	45g
Total Fat	5g	Carbohydrate	9g
Saturated Fat	1g	Cholesterol	120mg
Sodium	585mg	Fiber	0g

EXCHANGES: 6 Very Lean Meat

SAVORY BAKED LEMON-CHICKEN

1. 6 (6 oz.) Chicken Breasts (boneless, skinless)
2. 1 Teaspoon Garlic Salt
3. 2 Tablespoons Lemon Juice
4. 1/4 Cup Fat Free Margarine (melted)

Rub chicken with garlic salt and lemon juice. Place in baking dish and pour margarine over chicken. Bake at 350 degrees for 1 hour, basting often.
6 Servings.

SERVING SIZE - ONE

Calorie	289	Protein	53g
Total Fat	6g	Carbohydrate	1g
Saturated Fat	2g	Cholesterol	146mg
Sodium	528mg	Fiber	0g

EXCHANGES: 6 Very Lean Meat

CHERRY CHICKEN

1. 4 (6 oz.) Chicken Breasts (boneless, skinless)
2. 1 Tablespoon Lemon Juice
3. 1/3 Cup Cherry Preserves
4. Dash Ground Allspice

Pat chicken dry and place on rack of broiler pan. Broil 4-inches from heat for 6 minutes. Brush with lemon juice. Turn chicken over and brush with remaining juice and broil 6-9 minutes longer or until tender and no longer pink. In small saucepan heat cherry preserves and allspice. Spoon over chicken breasts and serve. 4 Servings.

SERVING SIZE - ONE

Calorie	311	Protein	54g
Total Fat	6g	Carbohydrate	7g
Saturated Fat	2g	Cholesterol	146mg
Sodium	128mg	Fiber	0g

EXCHANGES: 1/2 Fruit; 6 Very Lean Meat

CHICKEN ASPARAGUS ROLLS

LOW CARB

1. **4 (4 oz.) Chicken Breasts (boneless, skinless)**
2. **32 Asparagus Spears (tough ends removed)**
3. **2 Tablespoons Lemon Juice**
4. **6 Green Onions (chopped)**

Cut chicken breasts into 8 or 10 strips, each about l-inch by 5-inches long. Wrap each strip in a corkscrew fashion around 2 or 3 asparagus spears. Fasten with toothpicks. Place in a covered baking dish that has been sprayed with a nonstick spray. Sprinkle with lemon juice and onions. Cover and bake at 350 degrees for 30 minutes. Remove toothpicks. Serve hot or refrigerate until chilled and serve cold. 4 Servings.

SERVING SIZE - 8 SPEARS

Calorie	171	Protein	29g
Total Fat	3g	Carbohydrate	6g
Saturated Fat	1g	Cholesterol	73mg
Sodium	67mg	Fiber	0g

EXCHANGES: 4 Very Lean Meat; 1 Vegetable

MEXICAN CHICKEN

1. 4 (6 oz.) Chicken Breasts (boneless, skinless)
2. 1 Jar (16 oz.) Mild Thick Chunky Salsa
3. 1 Can (2 1/4 oz.) Sliced Black Olives (drained)
4. 1/2 Teaspoon Finely Chopped Garlic

Beat chicken breast to uniform thickness. Spray nonstick frying pan with olive oil flavored spray. Saute garlic over low heat. Add chicken and over low/medium heat cook until golden, turning once. Add salsa and cover. cook over low/medium heat 30-40 minutes. Good over rice. Top with olives.
4 Servings.

SERVING SIZE - ONE

Calorie	321	Protein	54g
Total Fat	8g	Carbohydrate	5g
Saturated Fat	2g	Cholesterol	149mg
Sodium	1083mg	Fiber	2g

EXCHANGES: 6 Very Lean Meat

CROCK POT CHICKEN

1. 4 (5 oz.) Chicken Breasts (boneless, skinless)
2. 1 Small Cabbage (quartered)
3. 1 Pound Package of Mini Carrots
4. 2 Large Cans (14 1/2 oz.) Mexican Flavored
    Stewed Tomatoes

Place above ingredients in crock pot. Cover and cook on low 6-7 hours. 4 Servings.

SERVING SIZE - ONE CUP

Calorie	323	Protein	47g
Total Fat	6g	Carbohydrate	21g
Saturated Fat	2g	Cholesterol	122mg
Sodium	493mg	Fiber	5g

EXCHANGES: 6 Very Lean Meat; 4 Vegetables

CHICKEN SOUR CREAM

1. 4 (3 oz.) Chicken Breasts
2. 1 Cup (8 oz.) Fat Free Sour Cream
3. 1 Package Dry Onion Soup Mix
4. 1/2 Cup Skim Milk

Mix sour cream, soup and milk and pour over
chicken breasts. Cover and bake at 350 degrees for
1 1/2 hours. 4 Servings.

SERVING SIZE - ONE

Calorie	185	Protein	34g
Total Fat	3g	Carbohydrate	4g
Saturated Fat	1g	Cholesterol	74mg
Sodium	153mg	Fiber	0g

EXCHANGES: 4 1/2 Very Lean Meat

TANGY CHICKEN

1. 4 (3 oz.) Chicken Breasts (skinless, boneless)
2. 1/2 Cup Onion (sliced)
3. 1/2 Cup Heinz 57 Sauce
4. 1/2 Cup Water

In skillet sprayed with nonstick spray, brown chicken and onion until breasts are not pink in the middle and onions are translucent. Combine sauce and water and pour over chicken. Cover and simmer for 40 minutes or until chicken is tender. Baste occasionally. Remove cover last 10 minutes of cooking. Spoon sauce over chicken and serve.
4 Servings.

SERVING SIZE - ONE

Calorie	187	Protein	28g
Total Fat	3g	Carbohydrate	9g
Saturated Fat	1g	Cholesterol	73mg
Sodium	596mg	Fiber	0g

EXCHANGES: 1/2 Vegetable; 4 Very Lean Meat

FIESTA CHICKEN

1. 4 (3 oz.) Chicken Breasts (boneless, skinless)
2. 1/2 Cup Yogurt
3. 2 Tablespoons Taco Seasoning Mix
4. 1 Cup Fat Free Cheese Cracker Crumbs

Coat chicken breasts with yogurt. Combine cracker crumbs and taco seasoning. Dredge chicken in mixture. Place in baking dish sprayed with nonstick spray. Bake uncovered at 350 degrees for 1 hour.
4 Servings.

SERVING SIZE - ONE

Calorie	370	Protein	34g
Total Fat	16g	Carbohydrate	39g
Saturated Fat	6g	Cholesterol	74mg
Sodium	695mg	Fiber	0g

EXCHANGES: 4 Very Lean Meat; 2 1/2 Starches

ITALIAN MUSHROOM CHICKEN

1. **4 (3 oz.) Chicken Breasts (skinless, boneless)**
2. **2 Cups Fresh Mushrooms (sliced)**
3. **1 Cup Chopped Onion**
4. **1 Jar (14 oz.) Spaghetti /Mushroom/Onion Sauce**

In a skillet brown chicken in nonstick spray. Push to one side and saute onions and mushroom until tender. Stir in spaghetti sauce and cover skillet. Simmer for 25 minutes or until chicken is tender. 4 Servings.

SERVING SIZE - ONE WITH 1/2 CUP SAUCE

Calorie	268	Protein	30g
Total Fat	7g	Carbohydrate	20
Saturated Fat	1g	Cholesterol	73mg
Sodium	500mg	Fiber	1g

EXCHANGES: 1 1/2 Vegetables; 1 Starch; 4 Very Lean Meat; 1 Fat

ONION RING CHICKEN

1. 4 (3 oz.) Chicken Breasts (skinless, boneless)
2. 1/4 Cup Fat Free Margarine
3. 4 Tablespoons Worcestershire Sauce
4. 1 Can (2.5 oz.) Fried Onion Rings (crushed)

Flatten each breast, season to taste. Combine margarine and Worcestershire sauce. Dredge chicken in margarine mixture, then crushed onion rings. Arrange on baking pan that has been sprayed with nonstick spray. Top with any remaining margarine mixture. Bake at 350 degrees for 45 minutes or until tender. 4 Servings.

SERVING SIZE - ONE

Calorie	228	Protein	29g
Total Fat	4g	Carbohydrate	17g
Saturated Fat	1g	Cholesterol	73mg
Sodium	432mg	Fiber	1g

EXCHANGES: 1 Starch; 4 Very Lean Meat; 1/2 Fat

CHICKEN MARSALA

1. 6 (3 oz.) Chicken Breasts (skinless, boneless)
2. 1 Clove Garlic (chopped)
3. 2 Cups Fresh Mushrooms (sliced)
4. 1/2 Cup Marsala Wine

Pound chicken until very thin and double the size. Saute the garlic and mushrooms in a large skillet sprayed with nonstick spray, over medium heat for 3 minutes. Remove mushrooms. Cook chicken 5 minutes on each side. Remove chicken and keep warm. Add mushrooms and Marsala Wine to the pan and heat for 1 minute. Place chicken on serving plate and pour mushrooms and juices over.
6 Servings.

SERVING SIZE - ONE

Calorie	163	Protein	27g
Total Fat	3g	Carbohydrate	2
Saturated Fat	1g	Cholesterol	73mg
Sodium	77mg	Fiber	0g

EXCHANGES: 1/2 Vegetable; 4 Very Lean Meat

LIME CHICKEN

1. 6 (3 oz.) Chicken Breast (skinless, boneless)
2. 2 Cloves Garlic (chopped)
3. 2 Tablespoons Cilantro
4. 1 1/2 Cups Lime Juice

Pour lime juice into a plastic container. Add garlic and cilantro. Add chicken and coat well. Chill for 1 hour or overnight. Place chicken on broiler pan and broil 6 inches from heat for 7-8 minutes on each side. 6 Servings.

SERVING SIZE - ONE

Calorie	160	Protein	27g
Total Fat	3g	Carbohydrate	6
Saturated Fat	1g	Cholesterol	73mg
Sodium	64mg	Fiber	0g

EXCHANGES: 1/2 Fruit; 4 Very Lean Meat

OPEN FACED CHICKEN CORDON BLEU

1. 4 (3 oz.) Chicken Breast (skinless, boneless)
2. 1 Tablespoon Fat Free Margarine
3. 4 Slices Fat Free Turkey Ham
4. 4 Slices Lowfat Swiss Cheese

Pound chicken breasts to flatten. Melt margarine in nonstick skillet over medium heat. Cook chicken 1 minute on each side. Place in square pan. Top each breast with a slice of ham. Pour pan drippings over chicken. Cover with tin foil and bake at 375 degrees for 25 minutes. Uncover and add a slice of cheese over each chicken breast. Cover and bake for an additional 5 minutes. 4 Servings.

SERVING SIZE - ONE

Calorie	276	Protein	41g
Total Fat	11g	Carbohydrate	2g
Saturated Fat	6g	Cholesterol	114mg
Sodium	443mg	Fiber	0g

EXCHANGES: 6 Very Lean Meat; 1/2 Fat

APRICOT LEMON CHICKEN

1. 4 (3 oz.) Chicken Breasts (skinless, boneless)
2. 1 Cup Water Packed Apricots
3. 2 Tablespoons Dijon Mustard
4. 3 Tablespoons Lemon Juice

Place chicken in baking pan. In a blender, blend apricots until smooth. Add mustard and lemon juice. Pour over chicken, cover and bake at 350 degrees for 40 minutes. Baste and bake uncovered 10 minutes more. 4 Servings.

SERVING SIZE - ONE

Calorie	170	Protein	28g
Total Fat	4g	Carbohydrate	5g
Saturated Fat	1g	Cholesterol	73mg
Sodium	243mg	Fiber	1g

EXCHANGES: 1/2 Fruit; 4 Very Lean Meat

SWEET ORANGE CHICKEN

1. **4 (3 oz.) Chicken Breasts (skinless, boneless)**
2. **1/3 Cup Orange Marmalade**
3. **1 Tablespoon Lemon Juice**

Place chicken in baking pan. Mix marmalade and lemon juice and spread on chicken. Cover and bake at 350 degrees for 40 minutes. Baste and bake uncovered for 5 more minutes. (NOTE: Do not use sugar free marmalade, the baking will make it taste bitter.) 4 Servings.

SERVING SIZE - ONE

Calorie	211	Protein	27g
Total Fat	3g	Carbohydrate	19g
Saturated Fat	1g	Cholesterol	73mg
Sodium	67mg	Fiber	1g

EXCHANGES: 4 Very Lean Meat

LEMONADE CHICKEN

1. 1 Can (6 oz.) Frozen Concentrate Lemonade
2. 1/3 Cup Worcestershire Sauce
3. 1 Teaspoon Low Sodium Soy Sauce
4. 4 (3 oz) Chicken Breasts (skinless, boneless)

Mix first three ingredients. Pour over chicken breasts and marinate in refrigerator for 1 hour. Place chicken and marinade in square pan. Bake uncovered at 350 degrees for 1 hour, basting occasionally. 4 Servings.

SERVING SIZE - ONE

Calorie	241	Protein	27g
Total Fat	3g	Carbohydrate	25g
Saturated Fat	1g	Cholesterol	73mg
Sodium	308mg	Fiber	1g

EXCHANGES: 1 1/2 Fruits; 4 Very Lean Meat

MUSHROOM CHICKEN

1. **6 (3 oz.) Chicken Breasts (skinless, boneless)**
2. **2 Cups Fresh Mushrooms (sliced)**
3. **1 Can Low Sodium, Low Fat Cream of Mushroom Soup**
4. **1/2 Cup White Table Wine**

Place chicken breasts in a 9x11-inch pan sprayed with nonstick spray. Place mushrooms on top of chicken. Mix soup and wine and pour over chicken and mushrooms. Cover with foil and bake at 350 degrees for 50 minutes. 6 Servings.

SERVING SIZE - ONE

Calorie	195	Protein	28g
Total Fat	5g	Carbohydrate	4g
Saturated Fat	1g	Cholesterol	73mg
Sodium	74mg	Fiber	0g

EXCHANGES: 4 Very Lean Meat; 1/2 Fat

PARMESAN CHICKEN

1. **4 (3oz.) Chicken Breasts (skinless, boneless)**
2. **1/2 Cup Fat Free Parmesan Cheese**
3. **2 Egg Whites**
4. **1/2 Cup Dry Seasoned Bread Crumbs**

Pound chicken breasts until double the size. Rub parmesan cheese into each side and pound it in well. Dip chicken in egg whites and press bread crumbs on both sides. Saute 3-5 minutes per side in skillet sprayed with nonstick spray. 4 Servings.

SERVING SIZE - ONE

Calorie	263	Protein	36g
Total Fat	7g	Carbohydrate	11g
Saturated Fat	3g	Cholesterol	83mg
Sodium	721mg	Fiber	0g

EXCHANGES: 1 Starch; 5 Very Lean Meat; 1/2 Fat

CHICKEN AND RICE DELUXE

1. 4 (3 oz.) Chicken Breasts (skinless, boneless, cut into cubes)
2. 1 Can Low Fat Cream of Chicken Soup
3. 1 Teaspoon Oregano
4. 2 Cups Instant White Rice

In skillet, brown chicken cubes with nonstick spray and oregano. Remove chicken from pan. Add soup and 1 1/3 cup water to skillet. Bring to a boil. Stir in rice and cooked chicken. Cover and cook on low heat for 5 minutes. 4 Servings.

SERVING SIZE - ONE

Calorie	270	Protein	31g
Total Fat	5g	Carbohydrate	23g
Saturated Fat	2g	Cholesterol	79mg
Sodium	664mg	Fiber	1g

EXCHANGES: 4 Oz. Very Lean Meat; 1 1/2 Starches; 1/2 Fat

SPICY TOMATO CHICKEN

1. 4 (3 oz.) Chicken Breasts (skinless, boneless)
2. 1 (4 oz.) Jar Mushroom Pieces
3. 1 (8 oz.) Can V8 Vegetable Juice
4. 1 Teaspoon Oregano

Place chicken breasts in baking pan sprayed with nonstick spray. Top with mushrooms. Pour V8 juice over chicken and sprinkle with oregano. Bake at 350 degrees, uncovered, for 1 hour. 4 Servings.

SERVING SIZE - ONE

Calorie	162	Protein	28g
Total Fat	3g	Carbohydrate	4g
Saturated Fat	1g	Cholesterol	73mg
Sodium	399mg	Fiber	1g

EXCHANGES: 1/2 Vegetable; 4 Very Lean Meat

CAJUN CHICKEN

1. **4 (3 oz.) Chicken Breasts (skinless, boneless)**
2. **1/2 Cup Corn Meal**
3. **1 Teaspoon Cayenne Seasoning**
4. **1/3 Cup Skim Milk**

Mix corn meal and cayenne pepper together and place in a saucer. Dip chicken in skim milk and then in the corn meal mixture. Place chicken in baking pan sprayed with nonstick spray. Bake uncovered at 350 degrees for 50 minutes. 4 Servings.

SERVING SIZE - ONE

Calorie	192	Protein	28g
Total Fat	3g	Carbohydrate	10g
Saturated Fat	1g	Cholesterol	73mg
Sodium	74mg	Fiber	1g

EXCHANGES: 1/2 Starch; 4 Very Lean Meat

CRUNCHY CORNFLAKE CHICKEN

1. 4 (3 oz.) Chicken Breasts (skinless, boneless)
2. 3 Cups Corn Flakes (crushed)
3. 1 Teaspoon Sage
4. 2 Tablespoons Skim Milk

Mix crushed corn flake crumbs with sage. Dip chicken in milk and press into crumbs, coating evenly. Place in a baking dish sprayed with nonstick spray. Bake uncovered at 375 degrees for 50-55 minutes. 4 Servings.

SERVING SIZE - ONE

Calorie	211	Protein	28g
Total Fat	3g	Carbohydrate	15g
Saturated Fat	1g	Cholesterol	73mg
Sodium	278mg	Fiber	1g

EXCHANGES: 1 Starch; 4 Very Lean Meat

ZESTY CRISP CHICKEN

1. **4 (4 oz.) Chicken Breasts (boneless, skinless)**
2. **1 Cup Egg Beaters**
3. **1/4 Cup Low Sodium Soy Sauce**
4. **1 1/4 Cup Corn Flakes (crushed)**

Mix egg beaters and soy sauce. Dip chicken pieces in soy sauce mixture. Coat with corn flake crumbs. Place on nonstick baking sheet and bake for 1 hour at 350 degrees. 4 Servings.

PER SERVING – ONE

Calories	223	Protein	36g
Total Fat	4g	Carbohydrate	9g
Saturated Fat	1g	Cholesterol	91mg
Sodium	773mg	Fiber	0g

EXCHANGES: 1/2 Starch, 5 Very Lean Meats

OVEN FRIED CHICKEN

1. **6 (5 oz.) Chicken Breasts (boneless, skinless)**
2. **1 Cup Crushed Corn Flakes**
3. **1/4 Cup Buttermilk**
4. **1 Teaspoon Creole Seasoning**

Combine creole seasoning and corn flake crumbs. Brush chicken with buttermilk and roll chicken in crumb mixture. Place chicken in nonstick baking dish and bake at 375 degrees for 1 hour. 6 Servings.

PER SERVING – ONE CHICKEN BREAST

Calories	211	Protein	36g
Total Fat	4g	Carbohydrate	4g
Saturated Fat	1g	Cholesterol	98mg
Sodium	312mg	Fiber	0g

EXCHANGES: 5 Very Lean Meat, 1/4 Starch

HONEY MUSTARD CHICKEN

1. **4 (3 oz.) Chicken Breasts (skinless, boneless)**
2. **1 Tablespoon Lemon Juice**
3. **1/3 Cup Honey**
4. **1/4 Cup Dijon Mustard**

Place chicken breasts in a pan that has been sprayed with nonstick spray. Sprinkle chicken with lemon juice. Mix honey and mustard in small dish. Spoon half of the honey mixture over chicken. Bake covered at 350 degrees for 15 minutes. Turn chicken over and baste with remaining sauce. Uncover and bake for 30 minutes longer. 4 Servings.

SERVING SIZE - ONE

Calorie	227	Protein	28g
Total Fat	4g	Carbohydrate	18g
Saturated Fat	1g	Cholesterol	73mg
Sodium	422mg	Fiber	0g

EXCHANGES: 4 Very Lean Meat, 1 Starch

CHICKEN WITH A GLAZE

1. 4 (3 oz.) Chicken Breasts (skinless, boneless)
2. 1/2 Cup Fat Free Catalina salad dressing
3. 1/2 Package Onion Soup Mix
4. 1/2 Cup Water Packed Apricots

Place chicken breasts in a pan sprayed with nonstick spray. Mix salad dressing and soup mix together. In a blender, blend apricots until smooth. Add apricots to soup and salad dressing mixture. Pour sauce over chicken, reserving some for basting. Bake uncovered at 350 degrees for 1 hour, basting every 20 minutes. 4 Servings.

SERVING SIZE - ONE

Calorie	183	Protein	27g
Total Fat	3g	Carbohydrate	8g
Saturated Fat	1g	Cholesterol	73mg
Sodium	326mg	Fiber	1g

EXCHANGES: 1/2 Starch; 4 Very Lean Meat

OVEN BARBECUED CHICKEN

1. 4 Chicken Breasts (3 oz., skinless, boneless)
2. 1 Tablespoon Lemon Juice
3. 1/2 Large Onion (cut into rings)
4. 1 Cup Fat Free Barbecue Sauce

Place chicken breasts in a pan sprayed with nonstick spray. Sprinkle lemon juice over chicken. Place onion rings on top of chicken. Pour barbecue sauce over onion rings. Cover with foil and bake for 25 minutes at 350 degrees. Remove foil, baste and bake uncovered another 20 minutes. 4 Servings.

SERVING SIZE - ONE

Calorie	205	Protein	28g
Total Fat	4g	Carbohydrate	12g
Saturated Fat	1g	Cholesterol	73mg
Sodium	575mg	Fiber	1g

EXCHANGES: 4 Very Lean Meat; 1/2 Vegetable

CHICKEN DIJON

1. 4 (3 oz.) Chicken Breasts (skinless, boneless)
2. 1/2 Cup Fat Free Mayonnaise
3. 1/4 Cup Dijon Mustard
4. 1 Cup Dry Bread Crumbs

Combine mayonnaise and mustard. Coat chicken with mixture and roll into bread crumbs. Bake at 350 degrees for 1 hour. 4 Servings.

SERVING SIZE - ONE

Calorie	290	Protein	31g
Total Fat	5g	Carbohydrate	26g
Saturated Fat	1g	Cholesterol	73mg
Sodium	1032mg	Fiber	0g

EXCHANGES: 2 Starches; 4 Very Lean Meat; 1/2 Fat

COMPANY CHICKEN

1. **6 Chicken Breasts (skinned and boned)**
2. **1/4 Cup Sherry or White Wine**
3. **1/2 Cup Chicken Broth**
4. **1/2 Cup Grated Parmesan Cheese**

Place chicken in baking dish. Pour wine and broth on top of chicken. Sprinkle with parmesan cheese. Bake covered 45 minutes and uncovered 15 minutes. 6 Servings.

PER SERVING - ONE

Calories	196	Protein	31g
Total Fat	6g	Carbohydrate	1g
Saturated Fat	2g	Cholesterol	80mg
Sodium	283mg	Fiber	0g

EXCHANGES: 4 Very Lean Meats, 1/2 Fat

BAKED CHICKEN PARMESAN

1. **2 Pounds Chicken Breasts**
2. **1 Cup Cornflake Crumbs**
3. **1/2 Cup Grated Parmesan Cheese**
4. **1/2 Cup Fat Free Mayonnaise**

Combine crumbs and cheese. Brush chicken with mayonnaise and coat with crumb mixture. Place in nonfat sprayed casserole dish and bake at 350 degrees for 1 hour. 8 Servings.

PER SERVING - 4-5 OUNCE CHICKEN

Calories	248	Protein	38g
Total Fat	6g	Carbohydrate	8g
Saturated Fat	2g	Cholesterol	101mg
Sodium	439mg	Fiber	0g

EXCHANGES: 1/2 Starch, 5 1/2 Very Lean Meats

LEMON PEPPER CHICKEN

1. **2 Pounds Chicken Breasts**
2. **Fat Free Butter Flavored Spray**
3. **1/2 Cup Low Sodium Soy Sauce**
4. **Lemon Pepper**

Place chicken in sprayed baking dish. Spray chicken with butter spray. Sprinkle soy sauce and lemon pepper on each piece of chicken. Bake at 350 degrees for 1 hour. 8 Servings.

PER SERVING - 4-5 OUNCES CHICKEN

Calories	204	Protein	36g
Total Fat	5g	Carbohydrate	1g
Saturated Fat	1g	Cholesterol	96mg
Sodium	683mg	Fiber	0g

EXCHANGES: 5 Very Lean Meats, 1 Fat

CHICKEN CACCIATORE

1. 2 Pounds Chicken Breasts
2. 1 Medium Onion (chopped)
3. 1 Jar (14 oz.) Spaghetti Sauce
4. 1/2 Teaspoon Dried Basil

Brown chicken over low heat in nonstick skillet. Cook chicken 10 minutes each side. Remove chicken and sauté onion until soft. Stir in sauce and basil. Place chicken on top of sauce. Cover and simmer 20 minutes. 8 Servings.

PER SERVING – 3-4 OUNCES CHICKEN

Calories	239	Protein	36g
Total Fat	7g	Carbohydrate	6g
Saturated Fat	1g	Cholesterol	96mg
Sodium	354mg	Fiber	1g

EXCHANGES: 1/2 Vegetable, 1/2 Starch, 1/2 Fat, 3 Very Lean Meats

CONFETTI CHICKEN

1. 1 1/2 Cups Chicken (cooked and cubed)
2. 2 Cans (14 1/2 oz. each) Seasoned Tomatoes With Onions
3. 1 Green Pepper (chopped)
4. 2 Cups Rice (cooked)

In skillet, combine first three ingredients and season to taste. Simmer for 10-15 minutes. Serve over rice. 4 Servings.

PER SERVING – 1/2 CUP (4 OUNCES)

Calories	288	Protein	31g
Total Fat	4g	Carbohydrate	34g
Saturated Fat	1g	Cholesterol	73mg
Sodium	589mg	Fiber	4g

EXCHANGES: 3 Vegetables, 1 Starch, 4 Very Lean Meats

BROILED AND SPICY CHICKEN

1. 6 (5 oz.) Chicken Breasts (boneless, skinless)
2. 1/2 Cup Fat Free Italian Dressing
3. 1 Cup Tomato Juice
4. 1/2 Teaspoon Chili Powder

Combine dressing, tomato juice and chili powder. Pour over chicken and marinate for several hours. Broil for 30 minutes or until done, turning once and basting frequently. 6 Servings.

PER SERVING – ONE CHICKEN BREAST

Calories	205	Protein	36g
Total Fat	4g	Carbohydrate	3g
Saturated Fat	1g	Cholesterol	97mg
Sodium	509mg	Fiber	0g

EXCHANGES: 5 Very Lean Meats, 1/2 Vegetable

LEMON GARLIC CHICKEN

1. **4 (5 oz.) Chicken Breasts (boneless, skinless)**
2. **1 Clove Garlic (minced)**
3. **1/2 Cup Fat Free Chicken Broth**
4. **1 Tablespoon Lemon Juice**

Using non-stick skillet sprayed with cooking spray, slowly sauté garlic over low heat. Add chicken and cook over medium heat about 10 minutes or until brown on both sides. Add broth and lemon juice. Heat to boiling and then reduce heat. Cover and simmer 10-15 minutes, or until chicken is done. Remove chicken and keep warm. Cook or reduce remaining liquid in pan, around 3 minutes. Pour over chicken and serve. 4 Servings.

PER SERVING – ONE CHICKEN BREAST

Calories	194	Protein	36g
Total Fat	4g	Carbohydrate	0g
Saturated Fat	1g	Cholesterol	97mg
Sodium	149mg	Fiber	0 g

EXCHANGES: 5 Very Lean Meats, 1 Fat

CHICKEN BREASTS WITH MUSHROOMS

1. 6 (5 oz.) Chicken Breasts (boneless, skinless)
2. 1 Tablespoon Basil
3. 1/4 Pound Fresh Mushrooms (sliced)
4. 3 Tablespoons White Cooking Wine

On stovetop, place chicken breasts in non-stick skillet. Over low/medium heat brown chicken for 1-2 minutes. Add mushrooms, basil and wine and continue to cook for 30 minutes or until thoroughly cooked. Spoon sauce over breasts while cooking. 6 Servings.

PER SERVING - ONE CHICKEN BREAST

Calories	199	Protein	36g
Total Fat	4g	Carbohydrate	1g
Saturated Fat	1g	Cholesterol	97mg
Sodium	85mg	Fiber	0g

EXCHANGES: 5 Very Lean Meats

HONEY CHICKEN

1. **6 (5 oz.) Chicken Breasts (boneless, skinless)**
2. **1/2 Cup Honey**
3. **1/3 Cup Lemon Juice**
4. **1/4 Cup Soy Sauce**

Combine honey, lemon juice and soy sauce. Brush chicken with half of the mixture and bake at 350 degrees for 20 minutes. Brush with additional mixture and bake for an additional 35 minutes or until done. Baste frequently. 4 Servings.

PER SERVING – ONE CHICKEN BREAST

Calories	385	Protein	54g
Total Fat	6g	Carbohydrate	25g
Saturated Fat	2g	Cholesterol	146mg
Sodium	578mg	Fiber	0g

EXCHANGES: 1 1/2 Starch, 5 Very Lean Meats, 1 Fat

MEXICAN CHICKEN

1. 4 (5 oz.) Chicken Breasts (boneless, skinless)
2. 1 Cup Mild Thick Chunky Salsa
3. 1/2 Can (1 oz.) Sliced Black Olives (drained)
4. 1 Cup Water

Beat chicken breasts to uniform thickness. Spray nonstick frying pan with olive oil flavored spray. Sauté garlic over low heat. Add chicken and over low/medium heat cook until golden, turning once. Add salsa and cover. Continue to cook over low/medium heat 30-40 minutes. Top with olives. 4 Servings.

PER SERVING – ONE CHICKEN BREAST

Calories	302	Protein	54g
Total Fat	7g	Carbohydrate	2g
Saturated Fat	2g	Cholesterol	148mg
Sodium	637mg	Fiber	1g

EXCHANGES: 5 Very Lean Meats, 1 Fat

ITALIAN CHICKEN

1. 4 (5 oz.) Chicken Breasts (skinless, boneless)
2. 1/2 Cup Fat Free Italian Dressing
3. 1 Teaspoon Lemon Pepper
4. 1 Clove Garlic

Combine Italian dressing, lemon pepper and salt. Pour over chicken breasts and marinate for 2 hours or more in refrigerator. Remove chicken from marinade and bake uncovered at 350 degrees for 45 minutes. Broil for last 5 minutes. 4 Servings.

PER SERVING - ONE CHICKEN BREAST

Calories	298	Protein	54g
Total Fat	6g	Carbohydrate	3g
Saturated Fat	2g	Cholesterol	146mg
Sodium	546mg	Fiber	0g

EXCHANGES: 5 Very Lean Meats, 1 Fat

CHICKEN AND RICE

1. 8 (4 oz.) Chicken (boneless, skinless)
2. 2 Boxes (6.2) Uncle Ben's Wild Rice Mix
3. 1 Can (4 oz.) Sliced Mushrooms
4. 1 Can (11 oz.) Mandarin Oranges

Place rice in bottom of roaster with cover. Sprinkle with 1 of the seasoning packets in rice. Lay chicken over rice. Pour mushrooms and oranges with juice over chicken. Sprinkle top with second seasoning packet. Add water, according to package directions, to cover rice. Cover and bake at 350 degrees, about 2 hours. Remove cover for last 20 minutes. 8 Servings.

PER SERVING – ONE CHICKEN BREAST

Calories	306	Protein	32g
Total Fat	3g	Carbohydrate	35g
Saturated Fat	1g	Cholesterol	73mg
Sodium	589mg	Fiber	2g

EXCHANGES: 2 Starch, 5 Very Lean Meats

TASTY CHICKEN

1. **4 (5 oz.) Chicken Breasts (skinless, boneless)**
2. **1/3 Cup Tomato Juice**
3. **1/2 Teaspoon Garlic Powder**
4. **1/2 Teaspoon Oregano**

Pound chicken with meat tenderizer mallet until uniform thickness. Roll chicken breasts in tomato juice. Place chicken on foil in baking dish and sprinkle with garlic and oregano mixture. Bake uncovered at 350 degrees for 45 minutes. 4 Servings.

PER SERVING – ONE CHICKEN BREAST

Calories	218	Protein	40g
Total Fat	5g	Carbohydrate	1g
Saturated Fat	1g	Cholesterol	110mg
Sodium	165mg	Fiber	0g

EXCHANGES: 5 Very Lean Meats, 1 Fat

Fish

SHRIMP MARINARA

1. 1 Clove Garlic (minced)
2. 1 Tablespoon Canola Oil
3. 1 Can (1 lb. 12 oz.) Italian Style Tomatoes
4. 1 Pound Shrimp (shelled, deveined)

Saute garlic in oil until tender. Add tomatoes and cook until sauce thickens and tomatoes break up, about 20 minutes. Add shrimp and cook 5 more minutes. Serve over rice. 4 Servings.

SERVING SIZE - 3 OUNCES SHRIMP MARINARA

Calories	203	Protein	25g
Total Fat	6g	Carbohydrate	14g
Saturated Fat	1g	Cholesterol	172mg
Sodium	672mg	Fiber	2g

EXCHANGES: 2 1/2 Vegetables, 3 Lean Meat, 1/2 Fat

TEXAS BOILED BEER SHRIMP

1. **2 Pounds Unshelled Large Raw Shrimp (deheaded)**
2. **2 (12 oz.) Cans Lite Beer**
3. **2 Tablespoons Crab Boil Seasoning**

In large pot, bring beer to boil with seasoning. Stir in shrimp and cover. Return to boil and simmer for 5 minutes. Turn heat off and leave shrimp in hot beer for a few more minutes. Drain shrimp and serve immediately. Serve with lemon wedges. 6 Servings.

PER SERVING – 1/2 CUP SHRIMP

Calories	203	Protein	31g
Total Fat	3g	Carbohydrate	5g
Saturated Fat	0g	Cholesterol	229mg
Sodium	462mg	Fiber	0g

EXCHANGES: 4 Very Lean Meat

BROILED SHRIMP

1. 1 Pound Shrimp (cleaned, peeled)
2. 2 Tablespoons Olive Oil
3. 2 Tablespoons Minced Garlic
4. 4 Teaspoons Chopped Parsley

Combine olive oil, garlic and parsley. Roll the shrimp in mixture and broil until pink (about 5 minutes). 4 Servings.

PER SERVING – 3 OUNCE SHRIMP

Calories	194	Protein	24g
Total Fat	9g	Carbohydrate	4g
Saturated Fat	1g	Cholesterol	172mg
Sodium	185mg	Fiber	0g

EXCHANGES: 3 Very Lean Meat, 1 1/2 Fats

MARINATED GRILLED SHRIMP

LOW CARB

1. 2 Tablespoons Lite Soy Sauce
2. 1 Tablespoon Canola Oil
3. 1 Tablespoon Honey
4. 1 Pound Large Shrimp (peeled, deveined)

Mix soy sauce, oil and honey and pour over shrimp. Marinate at least one hour. Place on skewers and grill or broil 4-5 minutes until cooked through and browned. 4 Servings.

SERVING SIZE - 3 OUNCES SHRIMP

Calories	161	Protein	23g
Total Fat	5g	Carbohydrate	4g
Saturated Fat	1g	Cholesterol	172mg
Sodium	479mg	Fiber	0g

EXCHANGES: 3 Very Lean Meat, 1/2 Fat

BROILED COD

1. 2 Pounds Cod Fillets
2. 2 Tablespoons Onion (grated)
3. 2 Large Tomatoes (cut into small pieces)
4. 1 Cup Low Fat, Low Sodium, Swiss Cheese (grated)

Place fillets in baking dish that has been sprayed with nonstick spray. Sprinkle onion and tomatoes over fillets. Broil 10 minutes. Sprinkle with cheese and broil another 3 minutes. 6 Servings.

SERVING SIZE - 3.5 OUNCES FISH FILLETS

Calories	179	Protein	26g
Total Fat	5g	Carbohydrate	4g
Saturated Fat	3g	Cholesterol	146mg
Sodium	91mg	Fiber	1g

EXCHANGES: 1/2 Vegetable, 3 1/2 Very Lean Meat

BAKED COD VINAIGRETTE

1. **1 Pound Cod Fillets**
2. **3 Tablespoons Fat Free Vinaigrette Dressing**
3. **Paprika**
4. **1 Tablespoon Minced Chives**

In lightly sprayed shallow baking dish, arrange fillets and brush with salad dressing. Sprinkle with paprika and chives. Bake, uncovered at 450 degrees for 10-12 minutes or until fillets flake with a fork. 4 Servings.

PER SERVING – 3 OUNCE FILLET

Calories	100	Protein	20g
Total Fat	1g	Carbohydrate	1g
Saturated Fat	0g	Cholesterol	49mg
Sodium	219mg	Fiber	0g

EXCHANGES: 3 Very Lean Meat

SPANISH FISH

1. 1 (1 lb.) Fish (Snapper, Redfish)
2. 1 Bell Pepper (chopped)
3. 1 Red Onion (chopped)
4. 1 Can (14 1/2 oz.) Seasoned Tomatoes

Line shallow pan with foil leaving ample amount hanging over the edges. Pour 1/3 of the tomatoes onto the foil. Place fish over tomatoes. Sprinkle the bell pepper and onion over the fish. Pour remaining tomatoes over fish and loosely close up foil. Bake at 350 degrees for 20 minutes per pound or until fish is flakey. 4 Servings.

SERVING SIZE - 3 OUNCES FISH

Calories	150	Protein	25g
Total Fat	2g	Carbohydrate	9g
Saturated Fat	0g	Cholesterol	41mg
Sodium	486mg	Fiber	2g

EXCHANGES: 1 1/2 Vegetable, 3 Very Lean Meat

BAKED ORANGE ROUGHY

1. 1 Pound Orange Roughy Fillets
2. 1/4 Cup Lemon Juice
3. 1 Teaspoon Tarragon Leaves
4. 2 Teaspoons Dried Mustard

Place fillets in large casserole that has been sprayed with nonstick spray. Squeeze lemon juice over fillets. Sprinkle dried mustard and tarragon leaves over fish. Bake at 400 degrees for 25 minutes. 4 Servings.

SERVING SIZE -   2 1/2-3 OUNCE FISH FILLET

Calories	84	Protein	17g
Total Fat	1g	Carbohydrate	1g
Saturated Fat	0g	Cholesterol	23mg
Sodium	87mg	Fiber	0g

EXCHANGES: 2 1/2 Very Lean Meat

FISH DELIGHT

1. **4 Fish Fillets**
2. **1/4 Cup Light Soy Sauce**
3. **1/4 Cup Lemon Juice**

Place fillets in casserole dish sprayed with cooking spray. Mix soy sauce and lemon juice. Pour over fish. Bake at 350 degrees for 20 minutes and then place under broiler and broil for 10 minutes. 4 Servings.

PER SERVING - 3 OUNCE FISH FILLET

Calories	94	Protein	16g
Total Fat	3g	Carbohydrate	2g
Saturated Fat	1g	Cholesterol	54mg
Sodium	678mg	Fiber	0g

EXCHANGES: 2 Lean Meat

EASY CHEESY FISH FILLETS

1. **1 Pound Fish Fillets**
2. **1 Onion (thinly sliced)**
3. **1/4 Cup Fat Free Mayonnaise**
4. **1/4 Cup Fat Free Mozzarella Cheese (grated)**

Place fillets in a single layer in baking casserole that has been sprayed with nonstick spray. Spread with mayonnaise and sprinkle with cheese. Top with onions. Cover and bake at 450 degrees for 10 minutes. Uncover and bake 4-6 minutes more or until browned. 4 Servings.

SERVING SIZE - 3 1/2 OUNCES FISH FILLET

Calories	141	Protein	25g
Total Fat	1g	Carbohydrate	7g
Saturated Fat	0g	Cholesterol	52mg
Sodium	354mg	Fiber	1g

EXCHANGES: 1/2 Vegetable, 3 1/2 Very Lean Meat

ORANGE ROUGHY WITH RED PEPPERS

1. 1 Lb. Orange Roughy
2. 1 Small Onion (cut into thin slices)
3. 2 Medium Red Bell Peppers ((cut into strips)
4. 1 Teaspoon Dried Thyme Leaves

Cut fillets into 4 serving pieces. Spray heated skillet with nonstick spray. Layer onion and pepper in skillet. Sprinkle with 1/2 teaspoon thyme. Place fish over onion/ pepper layer. Sprinkle with remaining thyme. Cover and cook over low heat 15 minutes. Uncover and cook until fish flakes easily with fork (about 10 minutes). 4 Servings.

SERVING SIZE- 3 OUNCES FISH

Calories	107	Protein	18g
Total Fat	1g	Carbohydrate	6g
Saturated Fat	0g	Cholesterol	23mg
Sodium	86mg	Fiber	2g

EXCHANGES: 1 Vegetable, 2 1/2 Very Lean Meat

COMPANY HALIBUT FILLETS

1. **4 (4 oz.) Halibut Steaks**
2. **1/2 Cup Sugar Free Apricot Preserves**
3. **2 Tablespoons White Vinegar**
4. **1/2 Teaspoon Dried Tarragon Leaves**

Spray broiler pan rack with nonstick spray. Place fish steaks on rack and broil 4 inches from heat for 4 minutes. Turn fish and broil 4 minutes longer. Mix remaining ingredients and spoon onto fish. Broil 1 minute longer or until fish flakes easily with fork. 4 Servings.

SERVING SIZE - 3 OUNCE FISH FILLET:

Calories	123	Protein	20g
Total Fat	1g	Carbohydrate	10g
Saturated Fat	0g	Cholesterol	49mg
Sodium	86mg	Fiber	0g

EXCHANGES: 1/2 Starch, 3 Very Lean Meat

SWEET MUSTARD FISH

1. **1 Pound Cod**
2. **1/2 Cup Thick and Chunky Salsa**
3. **2 Tablespoons Honey**
4. **2 Tablespoons Dijon Mustard**

Arrange fish in baking casserole that has been sprayed with nonstick spray. Bake at 450 degrees, uncovered, for 4-6 minutes. Drain any liquid. Combine remaining ingredients and spoon over fish. Return to oven for 2 minutes to heat sauce.
4 Servings.

SERVING SIZE- 3 OUNCE FISH

Calories	129	Protein	21g
Total Fat	1g	Carbohydrate	7g
Saturated Fat	0g	Cholesterol	50mg
Sodium	443mg	Fiber	0g

EXCHANGES: 3 Very Lean Meat

SHRIMP KABOBS

1. 1 Pound Shrimp (peeled, deveined)
2. 2 Large Green Peppers (cut 1 inch squares)
3. 1 Pint Cherry Tomatoes
4. 1 (8 oz.) Bottle Fat Free Italian Salad Dressing

Combine all ingredients in shallow dish. Cover and marinate at least 3 hours, stirring occasionally. On skewers, alternate shrimp, green peppers, and cherry tomatoes. Place on broiler rack and brush with remaining dressing. Broil 4 inches from heat 5 minutes, turn once and baste with dressing. 4 Servings.

SERVING SIZE - 3 OUNCES SHRIMP

Calories	178	Protein	25g
Total Fat	2g	Carbohydrate	13g
Saturated Fat	0g	Cholesterol	172mg
Sodium	973mg	Fiber	3g

EXCHANGES: 1 1/2 Vegetables, 1/2 Starch, 3 Very Lean Meat

TARRAGON FISH

1. 1 Pound Fish Fillets
2. 1/2 Cup Plain Nonfat Yogurt
3. 1 Teaspoon Dried Tarragon
4. 1 Ounce Reduced Fat Mozzarella Cheese (grated)

Arrange fish in baking casserole that has been sprayed with nonstick spray. Bake at 450 degrees, uncovered, for 4-5 minutes. Drain any liquid. Mix remaining ingredients and spread over fish. Bake 2 minutes or until cheese is melted. 4 Servings.

SERVING SIZE - 3 OUNCES FISH

Calories	121	Protein	24g
Total Fat	1g	Carbohydrate	3g
Saturated Fat	0g	Cholesterol	51mg
Sodium	134mg	Fiber	0g

EXCHANGES: 3 Very Lean Meat

TANGY APRICOT FISH

1. 1 Pound Orange Roughy Fillets
2. 1/3 Cup Nonfat Yogurt
3. 3 Tablespoons Apricot Jam
4. 1 Tablespoon Lemon Juice

Arrange fish in baking casserole that has been sprayed with nonstick cooking spray. Bake in preheated oven at 450 degrees, uncovered, for 4-5 minutes. Drain any liquid. Combine yogurt, apricot jam and lemon juice and pour over fish. Bake for 2 minutes longer to heat sauce. 4 Servings.

PER SERVING – 3 OUNCE FISH

Calories	129	Protein	18g
Total Fat	1g	Carbohydrate	12g
Saturated Fat	0g	Cholesterol	23mg
Sodium	101mg	Fiber	0g

EXCHANGES: 1 Starch, 2 1/2 Very Lean Meat

LEMON BUTTER DILL FISH

1. 1 Pound Orange Roughy Fillets
2. 3/4 Cup Fat Free Lemon Butter Dill Sauce for Seafood
3. 1/4 Cup Red Bell Pepper (thinly sliced)
4. 1 Tablespoon Grated Parmesan Cheese

Brush both sides of fish with 1/2 cup dill sauce. Arrange fish in baking casserole that has been sprayed with nonstick cooking spray. Place red pepper slices on top of fish. Drizzle rest of dill sauce over tops of fish and peppers. Sprinkle with parmesan. Bake, uncovered, at 350 degrees for 20 minutes or until fish flakes easily with a fork.
4 Servings.

PER SERVING – 3 OUNCE FISH

Calories	133	Protein	20g
Total Fat	2g	Carbohydrate	7g
Saturated Fat	0g	Cholesterol	32mg
Sodium	186mg	Fiber	0g

EXCHANGES: 3 Very Lean Meat, 1/2 Starch

BROILED SALMON STEAKS

1. **2 (8 oz.) Salmon Steaks (halved)**
2. **Nonfat Butter Spray**
3. **1 Teaspoon Dried Marjoram**
4. **Freshly Ground Pepper**

Spray salmon with nonstick spray. Sprinkle with 1/2 marjoram and pepper. Spray broiler rack with nonstick spray. Broil steaks 4 inches from heat source until first side is lightly browned (5 to 8 minutes). Spray, turn, and sprinkle with remaining half of marjoram and pepper. Broil 5-8 minutes longer or until fish flakes easily with fork. 4 Servings.

SERVING SIZE - 3 1/2 OUNCES FISH

Calories	150	Protein	26g
Total Fat	5g	Carbohydrate	0g
Saturated Fat	1g	Cholesterol	43mg
Sodium	105mg	Fiber	0g

EXCHANGES: 3 1/2 Lean Meat

SPICY BAKED FILLETS

1. 1 Pound Fish Fillets
2. 3/4 Cup Fat Free Mayonnaise
3. 2 Tablespoons Tabasco
4. 1/2 Cup Pepperidge Farm Herb Stuffing
    (crushed)

Mix mayonnaise and tabasco together in a small
bowl. Place crumbs in a saucer. Spread mayonnaise
mixture on both sides of fish and press fillets into
crumbs. Bake on a sprayed nonstick dish at 375
degrees for 30 minutes (or until fish flakes easily
when tested with fork). 4 Servings.

SERVING SIZE - 3 OUNCES FISH

Calories	239	Protein	23g
Total Fat	2g	Carbohydrate	31g
Saturated Fat	0g	Cholesterol	49mg
Sodium	1022mg	Fiber	0g

EXCHANGES: 2 Starches, 3 Very Lean Meat, 1/4 Fat

SWEET ORANGE FILLETS

1. 1 Pound Fish Fillets
2. 3 Tablespoons Orange Juice
3. 1/2 Teaspoon Paprika
4. 2 Tablespoons Honey

Mix orange juice, honey and paprika in a small pan and simmer for 1 minute. Place fish fillets in a sprayed nonstick baking dish. Pour sauce over fillets. Bake at 400 degrees for 15-20 minutes (or until fish flakes easily when tested with a fork).
4 Servings.

SERVING SIZE - 3 OUNCES FISH

Calories	121	Protein	20g
Total Fat	1g	Carbohydrate	7g
Saturated Fat	0g	Cholesterol	49mg
Sodium	62mg	Fiber	0g

EXCHANGES: 3 Very Lean Meat

DILL FILLETS

1. 1 Pound Fish Fillets
2. 3 Ounces Fat Free Cream Cheese (softened)
3. 2 Fresh Lemons
4. 1 Teaspoon Dill Weed

Spread softened cream cheese over one side of fillets. Place fillets, cream cheese side up, on a sprayed non-stick 9-inch square pan. Thinly slice one lemon and place over top of fillets. Squeeze juice of other lemon over fish. Sprinkle top of fillets with dill weed. Cover tightly with foil and bake at 400 degrees for 15 minutes (or until fish flakes when tested with fork). 4 Servings.

SERVING SIZE - 3.5 OUNCES FISH

Calories	121	Protein	25g
Total Fat	1g	Carbohydrate	3g
Saturated Fat	0g	Cholesterol	53mg
Sodium	218mg	Fiber	0g

EXCHANGES: 3 1/2 Very Lean Meat

FISH WITH LIME

1. **1 Pound Fish Fillets**
2. **3 Fresh Limes**
3. **1/2 Cup White Wine**
4. **1 Teaspoon Basil**

Place juice of 2 limes, white wine, and basil in a plastic zipper bag. Add fish and coat with juice, wine and basil. Refrigerate for 30 minutes. Cook in sprayed nonstick skillet for 5 minutes per side (or until fish flakes easily when tested with fork). Squeeze juice of third lime over cooked fish.
4 Servings.

SERVING SIZE - 3 OUNCES FISH

Calories	120	Protein	20g
Total Fat	1g	Carbohydrate	2g
Saturated Fat	0g	Cholesterol	49mg
Sodium	63mg	Fiber	0g

EXCHANGES: 3 Very Lean Meat

PARMESAN FILLETS

1. **1 Pound Fish Fillets**
2. **1/4 Cup Plain Nonfat Yogurt**
3. **1 Teaspoon Dijon Mustard**
4. **1/4 Cup Parmesan Cheese (grated)**

Mix yogurt and mustard in a small bowl. Place fish in a sprayed nonstick baking dish. Spread top side of fish with yogurt mixture. Sprinkle with most of the parmesan, reserving some for serving. Bake uncovered at 400 degrees for 15 minutes (or until fish flakes easily with fork). Sprinkle with reserved parmesan to serve. 4 Servings.

SERVING SIZE - 3 OUNCES FISH

Calories	134	Protein	24g
Total Fat	3g	Carbohydrate	2g
Saturated Fat	1g	Cholesterol	55mg
Sodium	278mg	Fiber	0g

EXCHANGES: 3 Very Lean Meat

STUFFED FISH FILLETS

1. **1 Pound Fish Fillets**
2. **3/4 Cup Onion**
3. **1 Package (8 oz.) Herb Seasoned Stuffing**
4. **1 Tablespoon Dijon Mustard**

Cook onion in 2 tablespoons of water for 3 minutes. Mix in crumbs and turn off heat. Cover. Trim fillets so they are 2-inches wide. Spread with dijon mustard. Spread stuffing mix on each fillet. Roll up, enclosing stuffing. Place each roll-up in a muffin cup that been sprayed with nonstick spray. Sprinkle with any left over stuffing. Bake at 400 degrees for 18 minutes. 4 Servings.

SERVING SIZE - 3 1/2 OUNCES FISH

Calories	349	Protein	30g
Total Fat	4g	Carbohydrate	47g
Saturated Fat	1g	Cholesterol	41mg
Sodium	920mg	Fiber	1g

EXCHANGES: 1/2 Vegetable, 3 Starches, 3 1/2 Very Lean Meats, 1/2 Fat

GAZPACHO FILLETS

1. 1 Pound Fish Fillets
2. 1 Cup Roma Tomatoes (chopped)
3. 1/2 Cup Green Onions (chopped)
4. 1 Teaspoon Garlic Powder

Place fish in a sprayed nonstick baking dish. Mix next 3 ingredients in small bowl. Spread on fish fillets. Bake at 400 degrees uncovered for 20 minutes (or until fish flakes easily with fork). 4 Servings.

SERVING SIZE - 3 OUNCES FISH

Calories	114	Protein	21g
Total Fat	1g	Carbohydrate	5g
Saturated Fat	0g	Cholesterol	49mg
Sodium	68mg	Fiber	1g

EXCHANGES: 1/2 Vegetable, 3 Very Lean Meat

ITALIAN FISH FILLETS

1. **1 Pound Fish Fillets**
2. **1/2 Cup Fat Free Italian Salad Dressing**
3. **2 Tablespoons Lemon Juice**
4. **1/2 Teaspoon Paprika**

Place fillets in a sprayed nonstick baking dish. Combine remaining ingredients and pour over fish. Bake at 375 degrees for 20 minutes (or until fish flakes easily when tested with a fork). 4 Servings.

SERVING SIZE - 3 OUNCES FISH

Calories	108	Protein	20g
Total Fat	1g	Carbohydrate	3g
Saturated Fat	0g	Cholesterol	49mg
Sodium	483mg	Fiber	0g

EXCHANGES: 3 Very Lean Meat

GARLIC SNAPPER

1. 1 Pound Red Snapper
2. 1/2 Cup Onion (chopped)
3. 1 Clove Garlic
4. 1 Can (16 oz.) Stewed Tomatoes

Spray skillet with nonstick spray. Saute onion and garlic for 30 seconds. Add tomatoes. Simmer for 10 minutes. Place snapper skin side down in a sprayed non-stick baking pan. Cover top of fish with sauce. Bake uncovered at 375 degrees for 30 minutes.
4 Servings.

SERVING SIZE - 3 1/2 OUNCES FISH

Calories	151	Protein	25g
Total Fat	2g	Carbohydrate	9g
Saturated Fat	0g	Cholesterol	41mg
Sodium	361mg	Fiber	1g

EXCHANGES: 1 1/2 Vegetables, 3 1/2 Very Lean Meat

GRILLED TUNA STEAKS

1. 4 (3 oz.) Tuna Steaks
2. 1 Cup Prepared Fat Free Italian Salad Dressing
3. 2 Teaspoons Fresh Ground Pepper
4. 1 Lemon

Place steaks in casserole. Pour dressing over tuna.
Cover and refrigerate for 1 hour, turning once.
Remove steaks from marinade and sprinkle pepper
on both sides. Grill or broil 5 minutes on each side.
Squeeze lemon over steaks and serve. 4 Servings.

PER SERVING – 3 OUNCE FISH

Calories	126	Protein	20g
Total Fat	1g	Carbohydrate	7g
Saturated Fat	0g	Cholesterol	38mg
Sodium	872mg	Fiber	0g

EXCHANGES: 1/2 Starch, 3 Very Lean Meat

SCALLOP KABOBS

1. 1 Pound Fresh Sea Scallops
2. 2 Large Green Peppers (cut 1-inch squares)
3. 1 Pint Cherry Tomatoes
4. 1 (8 oz.) Bottle Fat Free Italian Salad Dressing

Combine all ingredients in shallow dish lightly spray with cooking spray. Cover and marinate at least 3 hours, stirring occasionally. On skewers, alternate scallops, green peppers, and cherry tomatoes. Place on broiler rack and brush with dressing. Broil 4-inches from heat 5 minutes, turn and baste with dressing. 4 Servings.

PER SERVING – 1 SKEWER

Calories	175	Protein	21g
Total Fat	1g	Carbohydrate	19g
Saturated Fat	0g	Cholesterol	38mg
Sodium	987mg	Fiber	3g

EXCHANGES: 1/2 Starch, 2 1/2 Very Lean Meat, 2 1/2 Vegetables

SEASONED ORANGE ROUGHY

1. **1 Pound Orange Roughy**
2. **1 Teaspoon Thyme**
3. **1 Teaspoon Basil**
4. **1 1/2 Tablespoons Olive Oil**

Preheat oven to 350 degrees. In a small bowl, combine thyme, basil and oil into a smooth paste. Rub into each piece of fish. Place fish in a ovenproof glass baking dish sprayed with nonstick spray and bake uncovered until cooked through, about 30 minutes, depending on thickness. Place on serving platter and serve hot. 4 Servings.

SERVING SIZE - 3 OUNCES FISH

Calories	125	Protein	17g
Total Fat	6g	Carbohydrate	0g
Saturated Fat	1g	Cholesterol	23mg
Sodium	84mg	Fiber	1g

EXCHANGES: 1 Fat (monounsaturated), 2 1/2 Very Lean Meat

DIJON SALMON

1. **3 Salmon Fillets**
2. **1 Tablespoon Dijon Mustard**
3. **1 Teaspoon Dill Weed**
4. **1 1/2 Tablespoon Fat Free Mayonnaise**

Place salmon fillets skin side down in a sprayed nonstick baking dish. Coat top of fillets with mustard, then dill, then mayonnaise. Bake at 400 degrees for 25 minutes until golden brown.
2 Servings.

SERVING SIZE - 4 OUNCES FISH

Calories	198	Protein	31g
Total Fat	6g	Carbohydrate	3g
Saturated Fat	1g	Cholesterol	111mg
Sodium	394mg	Fiber	0g

EXCHANGES: 4 Very Lean Meat

HERBED SALMON STEAKS

1. 3 Packages (12 oz. each) Frozen Salmon Steaks
2. 1/4 Cup Lemon Juice
3. 2 Teaspoons Marjoram Leaves
4. 2 Teaspoons Onion Salt

Place frozen fish in casserole coated with cooking spray. Mix lemon juice, marjoram leaves and onion salt. Spoon on fish and bake at 450 degrees for 45 minutes. 6 Servings.

PER SERVING – 4 OUNCE FISH

Calories	210	Protein	34g
Total Fat	8g	Carbohydrate	1g
Saturated Fat	2g	Cholesterol	83mg
Sodium	809mg	Fiber	0g

EXCHANGES: 4 Lean Meat

CRUNCHY BAKED FISH

1. **1 Pound Fish Fillets**
2. **1/4 Cup Lemon Juice**
3. **1 Teaspoon Pepper**
4. **1 Cup Corn Flakes (crushed into 1/3 cup crumbs)**

Wash and dry fillets and cut into serving size pieces (3-4 oz.). Pour lemon juice into shallow bowl. Add fish and let marinate in juice 15 minutes. Drain fish. Coat with cornflake crumbs. Arrange in one layer in baking dish sprayed with nonstick spray. Bake for 10 minutes in 475 degree oven without turning.
4 Servings.

SERVING SIZE - 3 OUNCES FISH

Calories	124	Protein	21g
Total Fat	1g	Carbohydrate	7g
Saturated Fat	0g	Cholesterol	49mg
Sodium	134mg	Fiber	0g

EXCHANGES: 1/2 Starch, 3 Very Lean Meat

PARTY BAKED FISH

1. 1 Pound Orange Roughy Fillets
2. 1 Cup Party Mix (crushed into fine crumbs)
3. 1/2 Cup Low Fat Yogurt

Dip fillets into yogurt and then into the crushed party mix crumbs. Arrange in single layer in greased baking dish. Bake at 500 degrees for 15 minutes.
4 Servings.

PER SERVING – 3 OUNCE FISH FILLET

Calories	142	Protein	19g
Total Fat	3g	Carbohydrate	9g
Saturated Fat	0g	Cholesterol	24mg
Sodium	211mg	Fiber	0g

EXCHANGES: 1/2 Starch, 2 1/2 Lean Meat

CRISPY BAKED FISH

1. 1 Pound Orange Roughy Fillets
2. 1/3 Cup Finely Crushed Reduced Fat Cheese Crackers
3. 1 Teaspoon Fresh Parsley
4. 1/2 Cup Fat Free Catalina Salad Dressing

Preheat oven 400 degrees. Mix crackers and parsley. Brush both sides of fish with dressing. Coat one side of fish with cracker mixture. Place fish, cracker side up, on cookie sheet sprayed with nonstick cooking spray. Bake, uncovered, until fish flakes easily with fork, 10-15 minutes. 4 Servings.

PER SERVING – 3 OUNCE FISH

Calories	253	Protein	21g
Total Fat	5g	Carbohydrate	26g
Saturated Fat	1g	Cholesterol	23mg
Sodium	603mg	Fiber	1g

EXCHANGES: 1 1/2 Starch, 2 1/2 Very Lean Meat, 1 Fat

QUICK CRAB STIR-FRY

1. **8 Ounces Imitation Crab Meat**
2. **1 Package (10 oz.) Stir Fry Vegetables With Season Packet**
3. **1 Teaspoon Ginger**
4. **1 Tablespoon Balsamic Vinegar**

Spray a large nonstick skillet with cooking spray. Cook crab, vegetables and ginger for 2 minutes, stirring constantly. Mix sauce packet with 1/4 cup water and add to skillet. Heat for 1 minute. Add vinegar and heat for 1 more minute. 6 Servings.

SERVING SIZE - 1/2 CUP

Calories	59	Protein	5g
Total Fat	1g	Carbohydrate	8g
Saturated Fat	0g	Cholesterol	8mg
Sodium	328mg	Fiber	0g

EXCHANGES: 1 Lean Meat, 1/2 Starch

Pork

TEX MEX CHOPS

1. **4 Boneless Pork Chops**
2. **1 Cup Salsa**
3. **1 Bell Pepper (sliced)**
4. **1 Cup White Onion (sliced)**

Season pork chops to taste. In nonstick skillet sprayed with cooking spray, brown both sides of chops on medium high heat. Add salsa, bell pepper and sliced onion and lower heat. Simmer 30 minutes or until chops are thoroughly cooked. 4 Servings.

SERVING SIZE - 1 PORK CHOP

Calories	200	Protein	26g
Total Fat	7g	Carbohydrate	7g
Saturated Fat	2g	Cholesterol	62mg
Sodium	516 mg	Fiber	2g

EXCHANGES: 3 1/2 Very Lean Meat, 1/2 Vegetable

PORK CHOPS WITH RED CABBAGE

1. **4 Loin Pork Chops (cut 1-inch thick)**
2. **1 Large Onion (chopped)**
3. **1 Jar (15 oz.) Sweet/Sour Red Cabbage**
4. **1 Apple (quartered, cored, sliced)**

Brown pork chops in non stick skillet. Remove chops. Sauté onion until tender. Arrange chops over onions. Place cabbage and apple slices over top of pork chops. Cover and simmer for 30 minutes or until chops are cooked thoroughly. 4 Servings.

PER SERVING: ONE PORK CHOP

Calories	279	Protein	25g
Total Fat	7g	Carbohydrate	28g
Saturated Fat	3g	Cholesterol	61mg
Sodium	481mg	Fiber	1g

EXCHANGES: 2 Vegetables, 4 Lean Meats, 1 Fruit

MUSTARD-APRICOT PORK CHOPS

1. **1/3 Cup Light Apricot Preserves**
2. **2 Tablespoons Dijon Mustard**
3. **4 (3/4-inch) Pork Chops**
4. **3 Green Onions (chopped)**

Combine preserves and mustard in small saucepan. Heat and stir until preserves melt. Set aside. Place chops on lightly sprayed broiler pan. Broil 5 minutes. Brush chops with half of the glaze and turn. Broil 5 minutes longer. Turn and brush with remaining glaze. Broil 2 minutes. Garnish with green onions before serving. 4 Servings.

PER SERVING: ONE PORK CHOP

Calories	218	Protein	25g
Total Fat	8g	Carbohydrate	9g
Saturated Fat	2g	Cholesterol	61mg
Sodium	446mg	Fiber	0g

EXCHANGES: 1/2 Starch, 3 1/2 Medium Fat Meats

SAVORY BROILED PORK CHOPS

1. 4 (5 oz.) Lean Pork Loin Chops (3/4-inch thick)
2. 3 Tablespoons Dijon Mustard
3. 1 Teaspoon Dried Thyme
4. Freshly Ground Pepper

Spread half the mustard evenly over chops and sprinkle with half the thyme. Sprinkle with pepper. Broil 6 inches from heat 10 to 12 minutes. Turn chops and spread with remaining mustard and remaining thyme. Sprinkle with pepper. Broil second side until browned, around 10-12 minutes. 4 Servings.

PER SERVING: ONE PORK CHOP

Calories	231	Protein	32g
Total Fat	10g	Carbohydrate	1g
Saturated Fat	3g	Cholesterol	76mg
Sodium	440mg	Fiber	0g

EXCHANGES: 4 Very Lean Meats

ORANGE PORK CHOPS

1. **4 Lean Pork Rib Chops**
2. **1/3 Cup Light Orange Preserves**
3. **2 Tablespoons Dijon Mustard**
4. **4 Green Onions (chopped)**

In small saucepan mix marmalade and mustard and stir over medium heat until preserves is melted. Set aside. Place chops on broiler rack. Broil chops about 4 inches from heat for 6 minutes; turn and broil for 2 more minutes. Spoon half of the glaze over chops and broil 5 minutes more or until chops are no longer pink. In separate skillet sprayed with nonstick cooking spray, stir-fry the onions 2 minutes or until crisp-tender. Stir in remaining glaze and heat thoroughly. Serve over pork chops. 4 Servings.

PER SERVING: ONE PORK CHOP

Calories	218	Protein	25g
Total Fat	8g	Carbohydrate	9g
Saturated Fat	2g	Cholesterol	61mg
Sodium	446mg	Fiber	0g

EXCHANGES: 1/2 Starch, 3 1/2 Medium Fat Meats

BEST PORK TENDERLOIN

1. 1 1/2 Pounds Pork Tenderloin
2. 1 Teaspoon Black Pepper
3. 1 Teaspoon Rosemary Leaves
4. 1 Cup Barbecue Sauce

Rub tenderloin with pepper and rosemary leaves. Bake at 350 degrees for 1 1/2 hours. Slice and serve with warmed barbecue sauce. 6 Servings.

SERVING SIZE - ONE

Calories	210	Protein	25g
Total Fat	6g	Carbohydrate	14g
Saturated Fat	2g	Cholesterol	60mg
Sodium	626mg	Fiber	0g

EXCHANGES: 3 1/2 Very Lean Meat, 1 Starch

MARINATED PORK TENDERLOIN

1. 1 (1 1/2 Pounds) Pork Tenderloin Roast
2. 1 Tablespoon Sherry
3. 2 Tablespoons Lite Sodium Soy Sauce
4. 2 Tablespoons Brown Sugar

Combine sherry, soy sauce and brown sugar. Rub over meat and marinate overnight in refrigerator. Roast at 300 degrees until tender, 1 1/2 hours.
6 Servings.

SERVING SIZE - ONE

Calories	180	Protein	25g
Total Fat	7g	Carbohydrate	3g
Saturated Fat	2g	Cholesterol	66mg
Sodium	280mg	Fiber	0g

EXCHANGES: 3 1/2 Very Lean Meat

HONEY MUSTARD PORK TENDERLOIN

1. 2 (1 1/2 lb.) Pork Tenderloins
2. 1/2 Cup Honey
3. 2 Teaspoons Prepared Mustard
4. 1/4 Cup Brown Sugar

Mix honey, mustard and brown sugar. Spread over pork tenderloins and let marinate at least 2 hours in refrigerator. Roast at 350 degrees for 1 hour.
10 Servings.

PER SERVING: 3 1/2 OUNCES

Calories	206	Protein	25g
Total Fat	4g	Carbohydrate	14g
Saturated Fat	2g	Cholesterol	60mg
Sodium	94mg	Fiber	0g

EXCHANGES: 1 Starch, 3 1/2 Lean Meats

BAKED PORK TENDERLOIN

1. 1 (1 1/2 lb.) Lean Pork Tenderloin
2. Butter Flavored Non-Fat Spray
3. 2 Cups Canned Fat Free Chicken Broth
4. 1 Can (4 oz.) Mushroom Stems and Pieces

Brown meat in generous coating of butter flavored nonfat spray. Remove from skillet and place in casserole. Add a little flour to drippings and add chicken broth and mushrooms. Stir until heated and mixed. Pour over pork and bake at 350 degrees for 1 hour. 6 Servings.

PER SERVING: 4 OUNCES

Calories	168	Protein	27g
Total Fat	5g	Carbohydrate	1g
Saturated Fat	2g	Cholesterol	60mg
Sodium	418mg	Fiber	0g

EXCHANGES: 4 Lean Meats

PINEAPPLE PORK

1. 2 Pounds Lean Pork Tenderloin (cut in 1-inch cubes)
2. 1 Can (14 oz.) Pineapple Chunks (drain, retain liquid)
3. 1/4 Cup Vinegar
4. 1 Teaspoon Ginger

Combine above ingredients and simmer in nonstick skillet for 1 hour. Add pineapple liquid if needed. Chill, skim off fat and reheat. 8 Servings.

PER SERVING: 4 OUNCES

Calories	166	Protein	26g
Total Fat	5g	Carbohydrate	4g
Saturated Fat	2g	Cholesterol	60mg
Sodium	80mg	Fiber	0g

EXCHANGES: 1/2 Fruit, 3 1/2 Lean Meats

RAISIN SPICED PORK CHOPS

1. 1 Pound Lean Pork Loin Chops
2. 1/2 Teaspoon Pumpkins Pie Spice
3. 1/2 Cup Unsweetened Pineapple Juice
4. 2 Tablespoons (1 oz.) Raisins

Brown and heat pork chops in a nonstick skillet sprayed with cooking spray. Remove chops to heated platter. Combine remaining ingredients and cook over high heat, stirring constantly, until mixture is reduced to a few tablespoons. Pour over pork chops. 4 Servings.

SERVING SIZE - 1 PORK CHOP

Calories	202	Protein	25g
Total Fat	7g	Carbohydrate	8g
Saturated Fat	2g	Cholesterol	61mg
Sodium	68mg	Fiber	0g

EXCHANGES: 3 1/2 Very Lean Meat, 1/2 Fruit

SAUCY PORK CHOPS

1. **6 Lean Pork Chops**
2. **1 Cup Unsweetened Applesauce**
3. **1/4 Cup Lite Soy Sauce**
4. **1/8 Teaspoon Onion Powder**

Brown pork chops on both sides. Place in shallow casserole. Combine remaining ingredients and spoon evenly over chops. Cover and bake at 350 degrees for 45 minutes. Remove cover and continue baking 15 minutes longer or until chops are tender.
6 Servings.

SERVING SIZE - 1 PORK CHOP

Calories	187	Protein	25g
Total Fat	7g	Carbohdrate	5g
Saturated Fat	2g	Cholesterol	61mg
Sodium	483mg	Fiber	1g

EXCHANGES: 3 1/2 Very Lean Meat, 1/2 Fruit

DEVILED PORK ROAST

1. 1 (3 Pounds) Lean Pork Loin Roast
2. 2 Tablespoons Dijon Mustard
3. 1 Teaspoon Ground Thyme
4. Fresh Ground Pepper to Taste

Spread pork roast with thin coating of mustard. Sprinkle with thyme and pepper. Roast, uncovered, at 375 degrees for 1 1/2 hours. 12 Servings.

SERVING SIZE - ONE

Calories	169	Protein	25g
Total Fat	7g	Carbohydrate	0g
Saturated Fat	2g	Cholesterol	66mg
Sodium	130mg	Fiber	0g

EXCHANGES: 3 1/2 Very Lean Meat

PORK TENDERLOIN SUPREME

1. 2 (1 1/2 Pounds) Lean Pork Tenderloin
2. 1 Can Tomato Soup
3. 1 Package Dry Onion Soup Mix
4. 2 Tablespoons Worcestershire Sauce

Place tenderloins in center of large sheet of tin foil.
Mix remaining ingredients and spread over meat.
Seal securely in foil. Place in shallow pan and bake
for 2 hours at 325 degrees. Cut meat into l-inch
slices. Pour soup-gravy over slices of meat.
12 Servings.

SERVING SIZE - ONE

Calories	129	Protein	17g
Total Fat	5g	Carbohydrate	4g
Saturated Fat	2g	Cholesterol	44mg
Sodium	251mg	Fiber	0g

EXCHANGES: 2 1/2 Very Lean Meat

SAGE SEASONED PORK LOINS

LOW CARB

1. 1 Pound Lean Pork Tenderloin (cut into 1-inch slices)
2. 1/2 Teaspoon Dried Sage
3. 1 Small Onion (sliced and separated into rings)
4. 2 Apples (cored and cut into thin wedges)

Rub sage onto both sides of slices. Place slices in a large skillet sprayed with nonstick spray. Cook on medium-low heat for 5 minutes on one side. Turn and add onion and apples. Cook for 7 minutes more or until slices are thoroughly cooked. 4 Servings.

SERVING SIZE - ONE

Calories	197	Protein	26g
Total Fat	5g	Carbohydrates	12g
Saturated Fat	2g	Cholesterol	60mg
Sodium	80mg	Fiber	2g

EXCHANGES: 3 1/2 Very Lean Meat, 1/2 Fruit, 1/2 Vegetable

LEMON GARLIC ROAST PORK

1. 1 (3 Pounds) Lean Boneless Pork Loin Roast
2. 3/4 Teaspoon Grated Lemon Rind
3. 3 Garlic Cloves (minced)
4. 1 Can (14 1/2 oz.) Low Salt Chicken Broth

Trim fat from pork. Combine lemon rind and garlic and rub evenly over pork. Place pork in a casserole dish and add broth. Bake at 400 degrees for 30 minutes. Turn pork over and bake an additional 35 minutes. Discard broth and serve. 12 Servings.

SERVING SIZE - ONE

Calories	169	Protein	25g
Total Fat	7g	Carbohydrate	0g
Saturated Fat	2g	Cholesterol	66mg
Sodium	78mg	Fiber	0g

EXCHANGES: 3 1/2 Very Lean Meat

QUICKIE HAWAIIAN PORK

1. 2 Pounds Lean Pork Roast (cut in 1-inch cubes)
2. 1 Can (14 oz.) Pineapple Chunks With Juice
3. 1/4 Cup Vinegar
4. 1 Teaspoon Ginger

On stove top in large skillet, combine meat, pineapple with juice, vinegar and ginger. Simmer one hour covered. Serve over rice. 6 Servings.

SERVING SIZE - ONE

Calories	221	Protein	34g
Total Fat	6g	Carbohydrate	6g
Saturated Fat	2g	Cholesterol	80mg
Sodium	106mg	Fiber	1g

EXCHANGES: 5 Very Lean Meat, 1/2 Fruit

ROAST PORK IN MARINADE

1. 5 Pounds Lean Pork Tenderloin
2. 1 Can (15 oz.) Tomatoes (chopped)
3. 1/4 Cup White Vinegar
4. 1/4 Cup Water

Place roast in roasting pan. Mix tomatoes, vinegar and water and pour over roast and marinate overnight. Cover and bake at 350 degrees for four hours. 16 Servings.

SERVING SIZE - ONE

Calories	194	Protein	32g
Total Fat	6g	Carbohydrate	2g
Saturated Fat	2g	Cholesterol	75mg
Sodium	166mg	Fiber	0g

EXCHANGES: 4 1/2 Very Lean Meat, 1/2 Vegetable

HAWAIIAN BAKED PORK

1. 4 Pork Chops
2. 2 Cups Crushed Pineapple
3. 3 Medium Sweet Potatoes (peeled, sliced)
4. 2 Tablespoons Brown Sugar

Place pineapple with juice in large greased baking dish. Place sliced sweet potatoes over pineapple and sprinkle with brown sugar. Place pork chops on top of sweet potatoes. Bake covered 350 degrees for one hour, then uncover and bake at 450 degrees for 10 minutes. 4 Servings.

SERVING SIZE - ONE

Calories	296	Protein	27g
Total Fat	5g	Carbohydrate	36g
Saturated Fat	2g	Cholesterol	60mg
Sodium	91mg	Fiber	4g

EXCHANGES: 3 1/2 Very Lean Meat; 1 Fruit; 1 1/2 Starch

PEACHY PORK

1. **1 Pound Lean Pork Tenderloin (sliced)**
2. **1/2 Cup White Wine**
3. **2 Teaspoons Dijon Mustard**
4. **2 Tablespoons Peach Sugar Free Jelly**

Pound tenderloin slices to 1/4 inch thickness. Brown in sprayed nonstick skillet for 3-4 minutes. Remove and keep warm. Add remaining ingredients to skillet and heat until bubbling. Pour over tenderloin slices. 4 Servings.

SERVING SIZE - ONE

Calories	181	Protein	26g
Total Fat	5g	Carbohydrate	3g
Saturated Fat	2g	Cholesterol	60mg
Sodium	151mg	Fiber	0g

EXCHANGES: 3 1/2 Lean Meat

PORK STIR FRY

1. 2 Pounds Lean Pork Tenderloin (bite-sized pieces)
2. 1 Package (9 ounces) Frozen Carrots
3. 3 Cups Broccoli Florets
4. 1/3 Cup Sweet and Sour Sauce

Cook pork on medium high heat in a sprayed nonstick skillet, stirring constantly for 4 minutes. Add carrots and cook and stir for 2 minutes. Add broccoli and sauce. Cook, stirring constantly for 3-4 minutes until broccoli is crisp tender. Good served over white rice. 4 Servings.

SERVING SIZE - ONE

Calories	162	Protein	22g
Total Fat	4g	Carbohydrate	11g
Saturated Fat	1g	Cholesterol	45mg
Sodium	217mg	Fiber	4g

EXCHANGES: 3 Very Lean Meat, 1 1/2 Vegetables

POLYNESIAN PORK

1. 2 Pounds Lean Pork Tenderloin (cut into bite-size pieces)
2. 1 Can (20 oz.) Pineapple Chunks
3. 1 Bell Pepper (sliced)
4. 2 Tablespoons Lite Low Sodium Soy Sauce

In skillet sprayed with nonstick spray, brown pork cubes on medium high heat. Add remaining ingredients. Cover and simmer 45 minutes. Uncover, stir and simmer 15 more minutes. Good served over white rice. 4 Servings.

SERVING SIZE - ONE

Calories	162	Protein	20g
Total Fat	4g	Carbohydrate	14g
Saturated Fat	1g	Cholesterol	45mg
Sodium	373mg	Fiber	2g

EXCHANGES: 3 Very Lean Meat, 1 Fruit

PORK CASSEROLE

1. 2 Pounds Lean Pork (cut into 1-inch cubes)
2. 1 Large Can (16 oz. each) Sauerkraut (drained)
3. 2 Medium Onions (sliced)
4. 3 Cups Water

Brown pork in nonstick skillet and set aside. Spread 1/2 sauerkraut in 2 quart casserole sprayed with nonfat spray. Cover with 1/2 onion slices. Place pork on top. Layer remaining onions and sauerkraut on top of pork. Pour water over all, cover and bake. 6 Servings.

PER SERVING: 4 OUNCES

Calories	233	Protein	35g
Total Fat	6g	Carbohydrate	8g
Saturated Fat	2g	Cholesterol	80mg
Sodium	610mg	Fiber	3g

EXCHANGES: 1 Vegetable, 4 Lean Meats

Beef

CONEY ISLAND BURGERS

1. **1 Pound Lean Ground Beef**
2. **1/2 Cup Bottled BBQ Sauce**
3. **1/4 Cup Pickle Relish**
4. **1/4 Cup Onion (chopped)**

Combine ingredients and form into shape of hot dogs. Saute in skillet, turning until brown and cooked through. Place in hot dog buns and serve with mustard. 6 Servings.

SERVING SIZE - 1 HOT DOG SHAPED BURGER

Calories	183	Protein	17g
Total Fat	7g	Carbohydrate	12g
Saturated Fat	3g	Cholesterol	45mg
Sodium	309mg	Fiber	0g

EXCHANGES: 5 Lean Meat, 1 Fat, 1 1/2 Vegetable, 1/2 Starch

CREOLE PEPPER STEAK

1. 1 Pound Lean Beef Top Round Steak (cut 1-inch thick)
2. 2 Cloves Garlic (crushed)
3. 1 Teaspoon Dried Thyme
4. 1 Teaspoon Red Pepper

Combine garlic, thyme and red pepper, press evenly into both sides of steak. Grill 12-14 minutes for rare to medium, turning once. Cut steak diagonally into thin slices to serve. 4 Servings.

SERVING SIZE - ONE

Calories	140	Protein	26g
Total Fat	3g	Carbohydrate	1g
Saturated Fat	1g	Cholesterol	49mg
Sodium	64mg	Fiber	0g

EXCHANGES: 3 1/2 Lean Meat

ORANGE PEPPER STEAKS

1. 4 (4 oz.) Beef Tenderloin Steaks (cut 1-inch thick)
2. 1/2 Cup Orange Marmalade
3. 4 Teaspoons Cider Vinegar
4. 1/2 Teaspoon Ground Ginger

Combine marmalade, vinegar and ginger. Place steaks on rack in broiler pan and brush top of steaks with half of marmalade mixture. Broil 3-inches from heat for 10-15 minutes, turning once. Brush with remaining marmalade mixture after turning.
4 Servings.

PER SERVING - ONE STEAK

Calories	256	Protein	33g
Total Fat	11g	Carbohydrate	6g
Saturated Fat	4g	Cholesterol	97mg
Sodium	90mg	Fiber	0g

EXCHANGES: 4 1/2 Lean Meats

COMPANY BEEF TENDERLOIN

1. 6 (4 oz.) Beef Tenderloin Steaks
2. 8 Ounces Fresh Mushrooms (sliced)
3. 1 Large Clove Garlic (minced)
4. 1 Cup Cooking Sherry

In large nonstick skillet sprayed with cooking spray, sauté mushrooms and garlic for 4 minutes. Add sherry and cook until liquid is reduced. Stir frequently, set aside and keep warm. Broil tenderloin steaks for 5 minutes on each side. Arrange on platter and pour heated sherried mushroom sauce over steaks. 6 Servings.

PER SERVING - ONE STEAK

Calories	288	Protein	32g
Total Fat	11g	Carbohydrate	4g
Saturated Fat	4g	Cholesterol	95mg
Sodium	73mg	Fiber	0g

EXCHANGES: 4 1/2 Lean Meats, 1/2 Vegetable

SWISS STEAK

1. **2 Pounds Lean Top Round Steak**
2. **1/2 Cup Flour**
3. **1 Teaspoon Oil**
4. **2 Cans (14 1/2 oz. each) Stewed Tomatoes**

Flour steak and brown in oil. Remove from skillet and drain oil. Pour 1 can of tomatoes in skillet. Place steak on top and pour remaining can of tomatoes on steak. Cover and simmer for 1 1/2 hours. 6 Servings.

SERVING SIZE - ONE

Calories	257	Protein	37g
Total Fat	4g	Carbohydrate	17g
Saturated Fat	1g	Cholesterol	65mg
Sodium	433mg	Fiber	2g

EXCHANGES: 5 Lean Meat, 1/2 Starch, 1 1/2 Vegetables

MUSTARD ONION CHUCK ROAST

1. 2 Tablespoons Dry Mustard
2. 1 1/2 Teaspoons Water
3. 3 pounds Lean Chuck Pot Roast
4. 1/2 Cup Lite Soy Sauce

Blend mustard with water to make a paste. Cover and let stand for 5 minutes. Place tin foil in shallow baking pan. Place meat on foil. Stir soy sauce into mustard mixture, blending until smooth. Pour mixture evenly over roast. Fold and seal foil to cover roast. Bake at 325 degrees for 3 hours.

PER SERVINGS - ONE

Calories	348	Protein	27g
Total Fat	26g	Carbohydrate	1g
Saturated Fat	10g	Cholesterol	93mg
Sodium	579mg	Fiber	0g

EXCHANGES: 4 Lean Meat, 3 Fats

ROUND STEAK BAKE

1. 2 Pounds Round Steak
2. 4 Large Potatoes (peeled and quartered)
3. 2 Cans (6 oz. each) Mushrooms (reserved liquid)
4. 1 Package Dry Onion Soup Mix

Place steak on foil and sprinkle soup mix on steak.
Place potatoes evenly over steak and pour
mushrooms over potatoes and steak. Pour
mushroom liquid (add water if it doesn't make
1/4 cup liquid) over meat and vegetables. Wrap foil
tightly. Bake at 350 degrees for 1 1/2 hours.
6 Servings.

SERVING SIZE - ONE

Calories	313	Protein	40g
Total Fat	3g	Carbohydrate	30g
Saturated Fat	1g	Cholesterol	65 mg
Sodium	359mg	Fiber	4g

EXCHANGES: 1 1/2 Starches, 5 Lean Meat

BEEF STROGANOFF

1. 1 1/2 Pounds Lean Round Steak (cut in 1/4-inch strips)
2. 2 Tablespoons Dry Onion Soup Mix
3. 1 Can (6 oz.) Sliced Mushrooms
4. 1 Cup Fat Free Sour Cream

Brown round steak in skillet. Add soup mix and can of mushrooms with liquid to skillet. Heat until bubbly. Slowly add sour cream and cook until thoroughly heated. Good served with noodles.
6 Servings.

SERVING SIZE - ONE

Calories	161	Protein	31g
Total Fat	2g	Carbohydrate	3g
Saturated Fat	1g	Cholesterol	49mg
Sodium	219mg	Fiber	1g

EXCHANGES: 4 Lean Meat

SPANISH HAMBURGERS

1. 1 Pound Lean Ground Beef
2. 1 Large Onion (chopped)
3. 1 Can Healthy Tomato Soup
4. 1 Teaspoon Chili Powder

In large skillet, brown hamburger and onion. Drain off fat. Add soup and chili powder to hamburger mixture. Stir and simmer until hot. Serve over hamburger buns. 6 Servings.

SERVING SIZE -1/2 to 3/4 CUP

Calories	167	Protein	17g
Total Fat	8g	Carbohydrate	6g
Saturated Fat	3g	Cholesterol	45mg
Sodium	138mg	Fiber	1g

EXCHANGES: 1/2 Vegetable, 2 1/2 Lean Meat

CHILI MEAT LOAF

1. **2 Pounds Lean Ground Beef**
2. **1 Can (15 oz.) Chili With Beans**
3. **1/2 Cup Egg Substitute**
4. **1 Medium Onion (chopped)**

Combine ingredients. Shape into loaf and place into a greased shallow baking dish. Bake at 350 degrees for 1 1/2 hours. 8 Servings.

SERVING SIZE - 1/2 INCH SLICE

Calories	284	Protein	30g
Total Fat	14g	Carbohydrate	8g
Saturated Fat	5g	Cholesterol	76mg
Sodium	363mg	Fiber	2g

EXCHANGES: 1/2 Fat, 4 Lean Meat, 1/2 Starch, 1/2 Vegetable

MEXICAN MEATLOAF

1. 2 Pounds Lean Ground Beef
2. 1 Cup Picante Sauce (2/3 cup in loaf and 1/3 cup over top of loaf)
3. 1 Cup Bread Crumbs
4. 1/2 Cup Egg Substitute

Combine above ingredients, saving 1/3 cup picante sauce for top of meatloaf. Form into a loaf and place into an ovenproof pan sprayed with nonstick spray. Top with the remaining sauce. Bake at 350 degrees for 1 1/2 hours. 8 Servings.

SERVINGS SIZE - 1/2 INCH SLICE

Calories	279	Protein	29g
Total Fat	12g	Carbohydrate	12g
Saturated Fat	4g	Cholesterol	67mg
Sodium	420mg	Fiber	0g

EXCHANGES: 1/2 Starch, 4 Lean Meat

GROUND MEAT AND BEAN CASSEROLE

1. 1/2 Pound Extra Lean Ground Beef
2. 1/2 Cup Onion (chopped)
3. 2 Cans (16 oz.) Baked Beans
4. 1/4 Cup Catsup

Brown ground meat in skillet. Add onion and cook until tender. Add beans and catsup and heat thoroughly. 6 Servings.

SERVING SIZE - 1/2 CUP

Calories	154	Protein	12g
Total Fat	4g	Carbohydrate	19g
Saturated Fat	1g	Cholesterol	22mg
Sodium	411mg	Fiber	6g

EXCHANGES: 1 Starch, 1 Lean Meat, 1/4 Vegetable

SALISBURY STEAK

1. 1 Pound Extra Lean Ground Beef
2. 1/4 Cup Egg Beaters
3. 1 Medium Onion (chopped)
4. 1 Beef Bouillon Cube (dissolved in 1/2 cup water)

Mix beef, egg beaters and onion. Shape into patties and brown over high heat, drain off any fat. Pour in bouillon and simmer uncovered until desired doneness. 4 Servings.

PER SERVING - 1 PATTY

Calories	287	Protein	23g
Total Fat	19g	Carbohydrate	4g
Saturated Fat	8g	Cholesterol	76mg
Sodium	314mg	Fiber	1g

EXCHANGES: 1/2 Vegetable, 3 Lean Meats, 2 Fats

CABBAGE AND BEEF DISH

1. 1 Pound Extra Lean Ground Beef
2. 1 Medium Onion (chopped)
3. 3 Cups Cabbage (shredded)
4. 1 Can Tomato Soup

Brown ground beef and onion. Drain and season to taste. Spread in baking dish. Top with 3 cups cabbage. Pour tomato soup on top and cover. Bake at 350 degrees for 1 hour. 6 Servings.

PER SERVING - 1/2 CUP (4 OUNCE)

Calories	231	Protein	16g
Total Fat	14g	Carbohydrate	11g
Saturated Fat	5g	Cholesterol	51mg
Sodium	412mg	Fiber	2g

EXCHANGES: 1/2 Vegetable, 1/2 Starch, 2 Lean Meats, 1 1/2 Fats

MEAT AND POTATO DINNER

1. **4 Potatoes (peeled and sliced)**
2. **1 Pound Extra Lean Ground Beef (browned and drained)**
3. **1 Cup Green Peppers (sliced)**
4. **1 Can (28 oz.) Tomatoes (chopped)**

Layer above ingredients in order given. Cover and bake at 375 degrees for 45 minutes. Remove cover and continue baking until potatoes are done, approximately 15 minutes. 6 Servings.

PER SERVING - 1/2 CUP (4 OUNCE)

Calories	284	Protein	17g
Total Fat	13g	Carbohydrate	25g
Saturated Fat	5g	Cholesterol	51mg
Sodium	392mg	Fiber	3g

EXCHANGES: 2 Vegetables, 1 Starch, 2 Lean Meats, 1 1/2 Fats

VEGETABLE MEAT DISH

1. 1 Pound Extra Lean Ground Beef (browned, drained)
2. 1 Onion (chopped)
3. 4 Large Potatoes (peeled, sliced)
4. 1 Can (10 1/2 oz.) Vegetable Beef Soup

Brown ground beef and onions; drain. Place potato slices in lightly greased casserole. Spread ground beef and onions over potatoes. Pour soup over top. Cover and bake at 375 degrees for 45 minutes. Remove cover and continue baking until potatoes are done, approximately 15 minutes. 6 Servings.

PER SERVING - 1/2 CUP (4 OUNCE MEAT)

Calories	272	Protein	18g
Total Fat	14g	Carbohydrate	20g
Saturated Fat	5g	Cholesterol	52mg
Sodium	249mg	Fiber	2g

EXCHANGES: 1/2 Vegetable, 1 Starch, 2 Lean Meats, 1 1/2 Fats

BEEF GOULASH

1. **2 Pounds Lean Stew Beef**
2. **1 Large Onion (chopped)**
3. **1 Can (11.5 oz.) V8 Vegetable Juice**
4. **4 Cups Potatoes (cut into quarters)**

Brown meat and onions in nonstick skillet. Add V8 vegetable juice and potatoes. Cover and simmer 1 1/2 hours. Good served with noodles. 8 Servings.

SERVING SIZE - 3 1/2 Ounces Meat, 1/2 Cup Potatoes

Calories	286	Protein	28g
Total Fat	8g	Carbohydrate	24g
Saturated Fat	3g	Cholesterol	55mg
Sodium	215mg	Fiber	3g

EXCHANGES: 3 1/3 Lean Meat, 1/2 Vegetable, 1 1/2 Starch

FLANK STEAK AND SPINACH PINWHEELS

1. 1 1/2 Pounds Lean Flank Steak
2. 1 Package (10 oz.) Frozen Spinach (thawed, drained)
3. 1/4 Cup Grated Parmesan Cheese
4. 1/4 Cup Fat Free Sour Cream

Cut shallow diagonal cuts on one side of steak and pound to 3/8-inch thickness, Combine spinach, sour cream and cheese and spread on cut-side of steak. Starting at narrow end, roll up steak and secure with toothpicks at 1-inch intervals. Cut into l-inch slices (leaving picks in steak) and place pinwheels on broiler rack sprayed with nonstick spray. Broil 6 inches from heat, 7 minutes on each side. Remove picks and serve. 8 Servings.

SERVING SIZE - 3 OUNCES MEAT (1 PINWHEEL)

Calories	165	Protein	22g
Total Fat	7g	Carbohydrate	2g
Saturated Fat	3g	Cholesterol	37mg
Sodium	150mg	Fiber	1g

EXCHANGES: 3 Lean Meat, 1/2 Vegetable

SHERRIED BEEF

1. 2 Pounds Lean Beef (cubed in 1 1/2-inch cubes)
2. 2 Cans Cream of Mushroom Soup - Healthy Request
3. 1/2 Cup Cooking Sherry
4. 1/2 Package Dry Onion Soup Mix

Mix all ingredients in casserole and bake covered at 250 degrees for 3 hours. Good served with rice. 8 Servings.

SERVING SIZE - 3 1/2 OUNCE MEAT

Calories	207	Protein	27g
Total Fat	6g	Carbohydrate	6g
Saturated Fat	2g	Cholesterol	50mg
Sodium	94mg	Fiber	0g

EXCHANGES: 3 1/2 Lean Meat, 1/2 Fat

FLANK STEAK JOY

1. 2 Pounds Lean Flank Steak
2. 2 Tablespoons Lite Soy Sauce
3. 1 Tablespoon Sherry
4. 1 Teaspoon Honey

Mix soy sauce, sherry and honey and marinate meat in refrigerator 4 hours or longer. Remove the steak from marinade and place on broiler pan. Broil 6 minutes per side. Slice across the grain into thin strips and serve. 8 Servings.

SERVING SIZE - 3 1/2 OUNCE MEAT

Calories	143	Protein	25g
Total Fat	10g	Carbohydrate	1g
Saturated Fat	4g	Cholesterol	48mg
Sodium	225mg	Fiber	0g

EXCHANGES: 3 1/2 Lean Meat

BROILED FLANK STEAK

1. 1 1/2 Lbs. Lean Beef Flank Steak
2. 3/4 Cup Dry Red Wine or Cooking Wine
3. 1 1/2 Teaspoons Lemon Pepper
4. 1 Teaspoon Garlic

Combine wine, garlic and lemon pepper; pour over steak. Cover and marinate in refrigerator overnight. Remove flank steak from marinade. Coat broiler rack with cooking spray, and place flank steak on rack. Broil 3-4 inches from heat for 5-7 minutes on each side. Slice steak across grain into thin slices to serve. 8 Servings.

PER SERVING - 3 OUNCES MEAT

Calories	153	Protein	19g
Total Fat	6g	Carbohydrate	1g
Saturated Fat	3g	Cholesterol	34mg
Sodium	67mg	Fiber	0g

EXCHANGES: 3 Lean Meats

FLANK STEAK

1. 1 1/2 Pounds Lean Beef Flank Steak
2. 1/4 Cup Fat Free Margarine (melted)
3. 1 Teaspoon Garlic Powder
4. 1/2 Cup Dry Sherry

Combine sherry, margarine and garlic. Pour half mixture over beef and broil 3-inches from heat for 5-7 minutes. Turn, pour remaining mixture over beef and broil for 3 more minutes. Slice diagonally and serve. 8 Servings.

PER SERVING - 3 OUNCES MEAT

Calories	159	Protein	19g
Total Fat	6g	Carbohydrate	2g
Saturated Fat	3g	Cholesterol	34mg
Sodium	99mg	Fiber	0g

EXCHANGES: 3 Lean Meats

INDIAN CORN

1. 1 Pound Lean Ground Beef
2. 1 Can (16 oz.) Whole Corn (drained)
3. 1/2 Onion (chopped)
4. 1 Jar (12 oz.) Taco Sauce

In large skillet on stovetop, brown hamburger and onion; add corn and taco sauce. Simmer mixture for 5 minutes. Serve with baked tortilla chips.
6 Servings.

SERVING SIZE - 1/4 CUP MIXTURE

Calories	224	Protein	20g
Total Fat	9g	Carbohydrate	20g
Saturated Fat	3g	Cholesterol	45mg
Sodium	539mg	Fiber	2g

EXCHANGES: 1 Starch, 2 1/2 Lean Meats, 1/4 Vegetables

BBQ CUPS

1. **1 Pound Lean Ground Beef**
2. **1/2 Cup Barbecue Sauce**
3. **1 Can Refrigerator Biscuits**
4. **3/4 Cup Grated Fat Free Cheddar Cheese**

In skillet, brown meat, drain. Add barbecue sauce and set aside. Place biscuits in ungreased muffin cups, pressing dough up sides to edge of cup. Spoon meat mixture into cups. Sprinkle with cheese. Bake 400 degrees for 12 minutes. 12 Servings.

SERVING SIZE - 1 CUP/BISCUIT

Calories	208	Protein	15g
Total Fat	9g	Carbohydrate	17g
Saturated Fat	2g	Cholesterol	25mg
Sodium	540mg	Fiber	0g

EXCHANGES: 1 Vegetable, 1 Starch, 3 1/2 Lean Meat, 1 1/2 Fat

NEW YORK ROAST BEEF

1. **6-7 Pound Lean Eye Of Round**
2. **1 Teaspoon Canola Oil**
3. **1/2 Teaspoon Garlic Powder**
4. **1 Teaspoon Ground Oregano**

Rub oil all over roast. Combine garlic and oregano and rub over the oiled roast. Place in shallow baking pan with fat side up. Bake at 350 degrees for 20 minutes per pound. 12 Servings.

SERVING SIZE - 6 TO 7 OUNCES MEAT

Calories	500	Protein	49g
Total Fat	32g	Carbohydrate	0g
Saturated Fat	13g	Cholesterol	148mg
Sodium	122mg	Fiber	0g

EXCHANGES: 7 Lean Meat, 2 Fats

SAVORY SUNDAY ROAST

1. **2 Pounds Lean Chuck Roast**
2. **1/2 Package Onion Soup Mix**
3. **1 Cup Carrots (peeled)**
4. **2 Cups Potatoes (peeled and quartered)**

Place chuck roast in roasting pan with lid. Sprinkle onion soup mix on top of roast. Place carrots and potatoes around meat. Put 1/4 cup water into pan. Bake at 250 degrees for about 4 hours. 6 Servings.

SERVING SIZE - 4 OUNCES MEAT

Calories	284	Protein	33g
Total Fat	9g	Carbohydrate	17g
Saturated Fat	3g	Cholesterol	80mg
Sodium	163mg	Fiber	2g

EXCHANGES: 4 Lean Meat, 1 Starch, 1 Vegetable

STUFFED BELL PEPPERS

1. **4 Bell Peppers**
2. **1 1/2 Pound Lean Ground Beef**
3. **1 Package Sloppy Joe Seasoning Mix**
4. **1 Cup Tomato Sauce (No Salt)**

In nonstick skillet brown meat. Drain off remaining fat from pan. Add sloppy joe mix and tomato sauce. Simmer for 5 minutes. Fill peppers with meat mixture and place in a baking pan. Pour 1/8-inch water in baking pan around bell peppers. Cover with foil and bake at 350 degrees for 25 minutes. 4 Servings.

SERVING SIZE - 1 PEPPER

Calories	339	Protein	35g
Total Fat	14g	Carbohydrate	18g
Saturated Fat	5g	Cholesterol	87mg
Sodium	693mg	Fiber	4g

EXCHANGES: 1/2 Starch, 2 Vegetables, 4 1/2 Lean Meat

TATOR TOT CASSEROLE

1. 1 Pound Lean Ground Beef
2. 1/2 Cup Onion (chopped)
3. 1 Pound Frozen Tator Tots
4. 1 Can Low Fat Cream of Mushroom Soup

In skillet, brown onion and ground meat. Drain off any excess fat. Place hamburger meat in bottom of covered casserole dish. Place bag of frozen tator tots on top of meat. Pour can of mushroom soup on top of the tator tots. Cover and bake at 350 degrees for 30 minutes. 8 Servings.

SERVING SIZE - 1/2 TO 3/4 CUP

Calories	270	Protein	15g
Total Fat	14g	Carbohydrate	21g
Saturated Fat	6g	Cholesterol	34mg
Sodium	760mg	Fiber	2g

EXCHANGES: 2 Lean Meat, 1/2 Fat, 1/2 Starch

Pasta

GARLIC PASTA PRIMAVERA

1. 2 Cloves Garlic (chopped)
2. 1/2 Cup Low Salt Chicken Broth
3. 1 Package (12 oz.) Frozen Stir Fry Vegetables
4. Enriched Pasta (cooked and drained)

Saute garlic in nonstick skillet with cooking spray for 2-3 minutes. Add broth and vegetables. Let simmer for 15 minutes until most of the broth has cooked off. Mix in pasta. 4 Servings.

SERVING SIZE - 1 CUP

Calories	133	Protein	5g
Total Fat	1g	Carbohydrate	26g
Saturated Fat	0g	Cholesterol	0mg
Sodium	26mg	Fiber	1g

EXCHANGES: 1 1/2 Starches

MAMMA MIA PASTA

1. 1 Can (32 oz.) Italian Style Stewed Tomato
2. 1 Can (4 oz.) Mushroom Stems and Pieces
3. 2 Teaspoons Italian Seasoning
4. 1 Package (8 oz.) Enriched Pasta (cooked & drained)

Mix first three ingredients in medium saucepan. Simmer, uncovered, for 15 minutes, stirring occasionally. Serve over cooked pasta. 4 Servings.

SERVING SIZE - 1 CUP

Calories	117	Protein	4g
Total Fat	1g	Carbohydrate	26g
Saturated Fat	0g	Cholesterol	0mg
Sodium	687mg	Fiber	3g

EXCHANGES: 2 1/2 Vegetables, 1/2 Starch

HERBED PASTA

1. **1 Tablespoon Fresh Basil Leaves (chopped)**
2. **2 Teaspoons Olive Oil**
3. **2 Tablespoons Fresh Parsley (chopped)**
4. **1 Package (8 oz.) Enriched Pasta (cooked/drained)**

Mix all ingredients except pasta in a small bowl. Pour over cooked pasta. Toss to mix. Serve immediately. 4 Servings.

SERVING SIZE - 1 CUP

Calories	102	Protein	3g
Total Fat	3g	Carbohydrate	17g
Saturated Fat	0g	Cholesterol	0mg
Sodium	5mg	Fiber	1g

EXCHANGES: 1 Starch, 1/2 Fat

LEMON PASTA

1. 2 Tablespoons Fresh Parsley (chopped)
2. 2 Teaspoons Olive Oil
3. 2 Teaspoons Bottled Lemon Juice
4. 1 Package (8 oz.) Pasta (cooked and drained)

Mix all ingredients except pasta in a small bowl. Pour over cooked pasta. Toss to mix. Serve immediately. 4 Servings.

SERVING SIZE - 1 CUP

Calories	103	Protein	3g
Total Fat	3g	Carbohydrate	17g
Saturated Fat	0g	Cholesterol	0mg
Sodium	5mg	Fiber	1g

EXCHANGES: 1 Starch, 1/2 Fat

PASTA PRIMAVERA WITH PARMESAN

1. 1 Package (10 oz.) Frozen Mixed Vegetables With Seasoning Packet
2. 1 Tablespoon Butter Buds Granules
3. 1 Package (6 oz.) Enriched Pasta (cooked/drained)
4. 2 Tablespoons Parmesan Cheese (grated)

Place vegetables in a sprayed nonstick skillet. Stir fry for 2 minutes over medium heat. Add seasoning packet and butter sprinkles to 2 tablespoons water. Stir fry for 2 more minutes. Serve over pasta. Sprinkle with Parmesan. 3 Servings.

SERVING SIZE - 1 CUP

Calories	197	Protein	10g
Total Fat	4g	Carbohydrate	29g
Saturated Fat	0g	Cholesterol	7mg
Sodium	266mg	Fiber	3g

EXCHANGES: 2 1/2 Vegetables, 1 1/2 Starches, 1/2 Fat

SEAFOOD PASTA

1. 1/2 Pound Shrimp (peeled, deveined and cut-up)
2. 1/2 Cup Onion
3. 1 Can (16 oz.) New England Condensed Clam Chowder With 1 Can Water
4. 1 Package (16 oz.) Enriched Pasta (cooked & drained)

Saute shrimp and onions in sprayed nonstick skillet for 3-4 minutes. Add soup and salt and pepper to taste. Heat thoroughly. Serve over pasta. 4 Servings.

SERVING SIZE - 1 CUP

Calories	204	Protein	17g
Total Fat	3g	Carbohydrate	26g
Saturated Fat	0g	Cholesterol	88mg
Sodium	510mg	Fiber	2g

EXCHANGES: 1 1/2 Starches, 1 1/2 Very Lean Meat

VEGGIE PASTA BAKE

1. 1 Package (16 oz.) Frozen Mixed Vegetables (thawed)
2. 1 Package (8 oz.) Elbow Macaroni (cooked & drained)
3. 1 Jar (27 1/2 oz.) Spaghetti Sauce
4. 1 Package (8 oz.) Fat Free Mozzarella Cheese (grated)

In large bowl, combine vegetables, pasta and spaghetti sauce. Spray a 2-quart rectangular baking dish with nonstick spray. Spoon half of the pasta mixture in dish. Layer with half the cheese and add remaining pasta mixture. Cover with foil and bake at 375 degrees for 20 minutes. Uncover and sprinkle remaining cheese over casserole. Bake uncovered for 10 minutes more or until heated through. 6 Servings.

SERVING SIZE - 1 CUP

Calories	378	Protein	22g
Total Fat	8g	Carbohydrate	52g
Saturated Fat	1g	Cholesterol	7mg
Sodium	378mg	Fiber	6g

EXCHANGES: 2 Vegetables, 3 Starches, 2 Very Lean Meat, 1 Fat

PASTA WITH SPICY CLAM SAUCE

1. **1 Jar (30 oz.) Onion and Garlic Spaghetti Sauce**
2. **1 Can (12 oz.) Clams (reserving juice)**
3. **1/2 Teaspoon Cayenne Pepper**
4. **1 Package (12 oz.) Pasta (cooked and drained)**

Place spaghetti sauce, reserved clam juice and seasoning in medium pan. Chop clams and add to sauce. Heat almost to boiling. Serve over pasta. (hint: buy pasta sauce with oregano - it has a good flavor for this dish). 6 Servings.

SERVING SIZE - 1 CUP

Calories	243	Protein	9g
Total Fat	6g	Carbohydrate	37g
Saturated Fat	0g	Cholesterol	35mg
Sodium	669mg	Fiber	1g

EXCHANGES: 2 Starches, 1/2 Very Lean Meat

CREAMY CHEESY PASTA

1. 1 Jar (16 oz.) Marinara/Spaghetti Sauce
2. 1/2 Cup Grated Parmesan Cheese
3. 4 Tablespoons Fat Free Ranch Salad Dressing
4. 1 Package (12 oz.) Pasta (cooked and drained)

Combine marinara sauce, ranch dressing and cheese in a bowl. Add cooked pasta and mix together thoroughly. Put in microwave for 30 seconds or until completely heated. 6 Servings.

SERVING SIZE - 1 CUP

Calories	195	Protein	8g
Total Fat	7g	Carbohydrate	25g
Saturated Fat	2g	Cholesterol	7mg
Sodium	668mg	Fiber	2g

EXCHANGES: 1 1/2 Starches, 1/2 Very Lean Meat, 1/2 Fat

ITALIAN CHICKEN PASTA

1. 1 Package (16 oz.) Tri-colored Corkscrew Pasta (cooked and drained)
2. 1 Can (6 oz.) Water Packed Chicken (drained)
3. 4 Tablespoons Fat Free Italian Salad Dressing
4. 4 Ounces Grated Parmesan Cheese

Add chicken, salad dressing and cheese to cooked and drained pasta. Toss well. This dish is good hot or cold. 4 Servings.

SERVING SIZE - 1 CUP

Calories	343	Protein	28g
Total Fat	10g	Carbohydrate	35g
Saturated Fat	0g	Cholesterol	30mg
Sodium	764mg	Fiber	2g

EXCHANGES: 3 1/2 Starches, 2 1/2 Very Lean Meat, 1 1/2 Fats

Sauces

CHOCOLATE SAUCE

1. 2 Teaspoons Cornstarch
2. 1/4 Cup Cocoa Powder
3. 2 Teaspoons Vanilla Extract
4. 4 Packets Equal Sugar

Whisk corn starch and cocoa into 2 cups of cold water in a saucepan. Bring to a boil, whisking constantly, and cook over medium-low heat until thickened, about 2 minutes. Remove from the heat and stir in the vanilla extract and sweetener. Store in a screw-top jar in the refrigerator up to six weeks. (TO MAKE MOCHA SAUCE, SUBSTITUTE 2 CUPS STRONG COFFEE FOR THE WATER). 12 Servings.

SERVING SIZE - 3 TABLESPOON:

Calories	49	Protein	1g
Total Fat	2g	Carbohydrate	6g
Saturated Fat	0g	Cholesterol	1mg
Sodium	9mg	Fiber	0g

EXCHANGES: 1/2 Starch

GREEN CHILE SAUCE

1. 1 Can (8 oz.) Hot Green Chili Peppers
2. 1 Clove Garlic
3. 1 Can (16 oz.) Whole Tomatoes
4. 1 Teaspoon Salt

Blend chiles and garlic in blender until smooth. Add tomatoes one at a time and continue to blend. Add tomato liquid to make desired consistency. Stir in salt to taste. 32 Servings.

SERVING SIZE - 1 TABLESPOON:

Calories	5	Protein	0g
Total Fat	0g	Carbohydrate	1g
Saturated Fat	0g	Cholesterol	0mg
Sodium	97mg	Fiber	0g

EXCHANGES: Free Food

CHICKEN GRAVY

1. 1 Cup (8 oz.) Low Salt Chicken Broth
2. 2 Tablespoons All Purpose Flour
3. 1/4 Cup Skim Milk
4. 1/2 Teaspoon Pepper

Warm chicken broth in a saucepan over medium heat. Place flour and milk in a small bowl and whisk until smooth or place in a jar with a tight fitting lid and shake until smooth. Gradually stir milk mixture into chicken broth. Cook over medium heat, stirring constantly, until thick. Add pepper, reduce heat and continue to cook, stirring 5 minutes longer.
16 Servings.

SERVING SIZE - 1 TABLESPOON:

Calories	5	Protein	0g
Total Fat	0g	Carbohydrate	1g
Saturated Fat	0g	Cholesterol	0mg
Sodium	97mg	Fiber	0g

EXCHANGES: Free Food

ZIPPY FRUIT SAUCE

1. 1 Cup Raspberries (fresh or frozen)
2. 1 Cup Peaches (fresh or frozen)
3. 1 Tablespoon Bottled Lemon Juice
4. 6 Packets Equal Sugar

Puree all of the ingredients in a blender or food processor. If desired, strain through fine mesh strainer to remove seeds. Store in a tightly covered container in the refrigerator. Spoon over angel food cake or frozen sugar free, fat free yogurt.
32 Servings.

SERVING SIZE - 3 TABLESPOONS:

Calories	18	Protein	0g
Total Fat	0g	Carbohydrate	3g
Saturated Fat	0g	Cholesterol	0mg
Sodium	0mg	Fiber	0g

EXCHANGES: Free Food

QUICK HOLLANDAISE SAUCE

1. 2/3 Cup Liquid Egg Substitute
2. 1/4 Cup Bottled Lemon Juice
3. 1/2 Teaspoon Cayenne Pepper
4. 4 Teaspoons Butter Buds (Mix with 1 Cup Hot Water)

In a blender, combine eggbeaters, lemon juice and cayenne pepper. Blend at medium speed until mixed. Without turning off blender, pour in hot liquid butter buds in a slow steady stream. Continue blending until the mixture is smooth and thick. Mixture may be kept in top of double boiler over hot water for up to 10 minutes before serving to keep warm. Serve over vegetables, chicken or seafood. 6 Servings.

SERVING SIZE - 1/4 CUP:

Calories	17	Protein	3g
Total Fat	0g	Carbohydrate	1g
Saturated Fat	0g	Cholesterol	0mg
Sodium	83mg	Fiber	0g

EXCHANGES: 1/2 Very Lean Meat

GARLIC TOMATO MAYONNAISE

1. 1/2 Cup Fat Free Mayonnaise
2. 3 Tablespoons Tomato Sauce
3. 2 Cloves Garlic (chopped)
4. 6 Tablespoons Tomatoes (finely chopped)

Combine mayonnaise, tomato sauce and garlic. Cover and refrigerate at least 3 hours. Stir in tomato. Serve chilled as a sandwich spread, or warm over cooked vegetables. 16 Servings.

SERVING SIZE - 1 TABLESPOON:

Calories	9	Protein	0g
Total Fat	0g	Carbohydrate	2g
Saturated Fat	0g	Cholesterol	0mg
Sodium	113mg	Fiber	0g

EXCHANGES: Free Food

MOCK MAYONNAISE SPREAD

LOW CARB

1. 1 Teaspoon Prepared Mustard
2. 1/2 Teaspoon Low Sodium Soy Sauce
3. 2 Teaspoons Bottled Lemon Juice
4. 1 Cup Fat Free Cottage Cheese

Combine all of the ingredients in a blender. Blend until smooth. Serve chilled on your sandwiches in place of mayonnaise. 12 Servings.

SERVING SIZE - 1 TABLESPOON:

Calories	12	Protein	2g
Total Fat	0g	Carbohydrate	1g
Saturated Fat	0g	Cholesterol	1mg
Sodium	84mg	Fiber	0g

EXCHANGES: Free Food

BASIC WHITE SAUCE

1. **2 Cups Skim Milk**
2. **3 Tablespoons All Purpose Flour**
3. **1/2 Teaspoon Butter Buds Granules**
4. **1 Teaspoon Black Pepper**

Combine milk, flour and butter buds in a small saucepan. Heat, stirring constantly, until thickened. Season with pepper (salt optional). Use when you need a cream sauce as in macaroni and cheese or creamed chicken or tuna. 8 Servings.

SERVING SIZE - 1/4 CUP:

Calories	33	Protein	2g
Total Fat	0g	Carbohydrate	5g
Saturated Fat	0g	Cholesterol	1mg
Sodium	42mg	Fiber	0g

EXCHANGES: 1/2 Starch

TANGY SOUR CREAM

1. 1/2 Cup Plain Nonfat Yogurt
2. 1/2 Cup Fat Free Cottage Cheese
3. 1 Teaspoon Bottled Lemon Juice
4. 2 Packets Equal Sugar

Mix above ingredients in food processor or blender or beat with a mixer until smooth. Refrigerate in a covered container. This is a great substitute for whipped cream, mayonnaise or sour cream.
16 Servings.

SERVING SIZE - 1 TABLESPOON:

Calories	9	Protein	1g
Total Fat	0g	Carbohydrate	1g
Saturated Fat	0g	Cholesterol	0mg
Sodium	31mg	Fiber	0g

EXCHANGES: Free Food

SPICY TOPPER

1. **3/4 Cup Plain Nonfat Yogurt**
2. **2 Tablespoons Prepared Horseradish**
3. **1 Tablespoon Fresh Chives (chopped)**
4. **1/4 Cup Red Onion (chopped)**

Mix yogurt, horseradish, chives and onion together. Serve heated with roast beef or chilled for baked potatoes. 16 Servings.

SERVING SIZE - 1 TABLESPOON:

Calories	8	Protein	1g
Total Fat	0g	Carbohydrate	1g
Saturated Fat	0g	Cholesterol	0mg
Sodium	29mg	Fiber	0g

EXCHANGES: Free Food

FOUR MINUTE GRAVY

1. 1 Tablespoon Canola Oil
2. 2 Tablespoons All Purpose Flour
3. 1 Cup Skim Milk
4. 1/2 Teaspoon Onion Powder

Blend oil and flour in a non-stick sauce pan. Using a rubber spatula, slowly stir in cold milk. Mix until smooth. Add onion powder. Cook over medium heat, stirring until it thickens. Cooking time is about 3 minutes. Use this gravy instead of canned gravy, canned soups, pan drippings or cream sauces.
16 Servings.

SERVING SIZE - 1 TABLESPOON:

Calories	17	Protein	1g
Total Fat	1g	Carbohydrate	2g
Saturated Fat	0g	Cholesterol	0mg
Sodium	8mg	Fiber	0g

EXCHANGES: Free Food

ORANGE CREAM CHEESE GLAZE

1. 1 Package (8 oz.) Lowfat Cream Cheese
2. 1 Teaspoon Orange Extract
3. 3 Packets Equal Sugar
4. 1/4 Cup Skim Milk

Mix cream cheese, extract and sugar substitute and enough milk to make medium glaze consistency. Great served on sponge cake. 30 Servings.

SERVING SIZE - 1 TEASPOON:

Calories	19	Protein	1g
Total Fat	1g	Carbohydrate	1g
Saturated Fat	0g	Cholesterol	5mg
Sodium	54mg	Fiber	0g

EXCHANGES: Free Food

STRAWBERRY SAUCE

1. 1 Package (16 oz.) Frozen Unsweetened Strawberries (Thawed)
2. 1 Tablespoon Bottled Lemon Juice
3. 6 Packets Equal Sugar

Blend strawberries in a food processor or blender until smooth. Stir in lemon juice and equal sugar. Refrigerate until serving time. Great angel food topper. 32 Servings.

SERVING SIZE - 2 TABLESPOONS:

Calories	12	Protein	0g
Total Fat	0g	Carbohydrate	4g
Saturated Fat	0g	Cholesterol	0mg
Sodium	0mg	Fiber	0g

EXCHANGES: Free Food

Desserts

STRAWBERRY TRIFLE

1. 2 Packages (3.4 oz. Each) Sugar Free Instant Vanilla Pudding
2. 4 Cups Skim Milk
3. 20 Vanilla Wafer Cookies
4. 2 Pints (12 oz.) Strawberries (hulled and sliced)

Combine pudding mix and milk and beat. Pour half of pudding into 2 quart bowl or trifle dish. Top with vanilla wafers, then sprinkle with strawberries. Top with remaining pudding. Cover and refrigerate at least 4 hours or up to 24 hours. 16 Servings.

SERVING SIZE - 1/2 CUP

Calories	96	Protein	2g
Total Fat	1g	Carbohydrate	10g
Saturated Fat	0g	Cholesterol	4mg
Sodium	213mg	Fiber	0g

EXCHANGES: 1 Starch

CHERRY VANILLA TRIFLE

1. **1 Fat Free Prepared Angel Food Cake (torn into bite-sized pieces)**
2. **2 Containers (8 oz.) Fat Free Cherry Vanilla Yogurt**
3. **4 Containers Prepared Jello Sugar Free Vanilla Pudding Snacks**
4. **1 Can (20 oz.) Sweet Cherries (drained, water packed)**

Combine yogurt and pudding. Beginning with cake pieces, place a layer of cake with a layer of yogurt/pudding mix. Sprinkle with cherries. Repeat, ending with yogurt/pudding mixture. Cover and refrigerate. 12 Servings.

PER SERVING – ONE

Calories	196	Protein	7g
Total Fat	1g	Carbohydrate	41g
Saturated Fat	0g	Cholesterol	1mg
Sodium	212mg	Fiber	0g

EXCHANGES: 2 Starch, 1/2 Fruit, 1/2 Milk

ORANGE COCONUT BALLS

1. 3 Cups Finely Crushed Vanilla Wafers
2. 2 Cups Flaked Coconut
3. 1 Cup Pecans (finely chopped)
4. 1 Can (6 oz) Orange Juice Concentrate (thawed)

Combine ingredients and shape into bite sized balls. If desired, roll in crushed vanilla wafer crumbs. Refrigerate in airtight container. 20 Servings.

SERVING SIZE - 2 BALLS

Calories	244	Protein	3g
Total Fat	11g	Carbohydrate	34g
Saturated Fat	3g	Cholesterol	21mg
Sodium	87mg	Fiber	1g

EXCHANGES: 1/2 Fruit, 2 Starches, 1 Fat

RAISIN TREATS

1. **1/4 Cup Fat Free Margarine**
2. **1 Package (10 oz.) Marshmallows**
3. **1 Cup Raisins**
4. **5 Cups Rice Krispies**

Melt margarine over low heat in double boiler. Add marshmallows and stir until completely melted. Cook over low heat 3 minutes, stirring constantly. Remove from heat and add cereal and raisins. Stir until well coated. Pour and press mixture evenly into 9x13-inch cake pan sprayed with nonstick spray. Cut into squares when cool. 24 Servings.

SERVING SIZE - 1 SQUARE

Calories	88	Protein	1g
Total Fat	0g	Carbohydrate	21g
Saturated Fat	0g	Cholesterol	0mg
Sodium	83mg	Fiber	0g

EXCHANGES: 1/2 Fruit, 1/2 Starch

PINEAPPLE ORANGE FLUFF

1. 1 Package (3 oz.) Sugar Free Orange Jello
2. 1 Can (15 oz.) Water Packed Crushed Pineapple (undrained)
3. 2 Cups Buttermilk
4. 1 Container (8 oz.) Lite Cool Whip

Heat crushed pineapple and add orange jello. Stir until jello is dissolved. Cool about 15 minutes. Add buttermilk and cool whip. Stir until blended and refrigerate until firm. 10 Servings.

SERVING SIZE - 1/2 CUP

Calories	86	Protein	2g
Total Fat	4g	Carbohydrate	11g
Saturated Fat	0g	Cholesterol	2mg
Sodium	87mg	Fiber	0g

EXCHANGES: 1/2 Fruit, 1 Fat

STRAWBERRY/PEACH YOGURT PIE

1. 2 Cups Strawberry/Peach Yogurt Made With Aspartame
2. 1/2 Cup Low Calorie, Low Sugar Strawberry Preserves
3. 1 Carton (8 oz.) Lite Cool Whip (thawed)
4. Prepared Graham Cracker Crust

Combine strawberry preserves and yogurt in bowl. Fold in Cool Whip. Spoon into graham cracker crust and freeze. Remove and place in refrigerator for 30 minutes before serving. 8 Servings.

SERVING SIZE - 1 SLICE

Calories	262	Protein	4g
Total Fat	11g	Carbohydrate	36g
Saturated Fat	2g	Cholesterol	3mg
Sodium	240mg	Fiber	0g

EXCHANGES: 1 1/2 Starch, 3 Fat

ANGEL CAKE

1. 1 Package White Angel Food Cake Mix
2. 1 Cup Skim Milk
3. 1 Package (1 oz.) Milk Chocolate Sugar Free
   Instant Pudding Mix
4. 2 Cups (16 oz.) Lite Cool Whip

Prepare cake according to package directions for
tube pan. Split cake horizontally to make 2 layers.
Beat milk and pudding mix until well blended. Fold
in Cool Whip. Frost layers and top of cake
Refrigerate at least 1 hour before serving.
12 Servings.

SERVING SIZE - 1 SLICE

Calories	249	Protein	4g
Total Fat	5g	Carbohydrate	46g
Saturated Fat	0g	Cholesterol	1mg
Sodium	407mg	Fiber	0g

EXCHANGES: 2 1/2 Starches, 2 Fats

GINGERSNAP-BAKED PEARS

1. **1 Can (16 oz.) Unsweetened Pear Halves (drained)**
2. **12 Lowfat Gingersnaps (finely crushed)**
3. **2 Tablespoons Sugar**
4. **2 Tablespoons Fat Free Margarine (melted)**

Arrange pears, cut side up, in a 9-inch cake pan. Combine remaining ingredients. Spread over pears. Bake at 300 degrees for 20 minutes. Serve warm. 4 Servings.

SERVING SIZE - 1/4 OF PEAR

Calories	154	Protein	1g
Total Fat	2g	Carbohydrate	33g
Saturated Fat	0g	Cholesterol	0mg
Sodium	188mg	Fiber	1g

EXCHANGES: 1 Fruit, 1 Starch, 1/2 Fat

GINGERALE BAKED APPLES

1. **4 Large Baking Apples**
2. **4 Tablespoons Golden Raisins**
3. **4 Teaspoons Brown Sugar**
4. **1/2 Cup Gingerale**

Core apples without cutting through the bottom. Stand apples in baking dish just large enough to hold them. Place 1 tablespoon raisins and 1 teaspoon brown sugar in center of each apple. Pour gingerale into center. Bake at 350 degrees for 45 minutes, basting frequently, until apples are tender, but not mushy. Serve warm or chilled. 4 Servings.

PER SERVING – ONE APPLE

Calories	147	Protein	1g
Total Fat	1g	Carbohydrate	38g
Saturated Fat	0g	Cholesterol	0mg
Sodium	5mg	Fiber	3g

EXCHANGES: 2 Fruits, 1/2 Starch

OATMEAL MACAROONS

1. 2 Egg Whites
2. 1/3 Cup Sugar Free Maple Syrup
3. 1 Cup Rolled Oats
4. 1/2 Cup Grated Coconut

Beat egg whites until stiff. Combine syrup and oats in separate bowl and mix until well blended. Add coconut. Fold in beaten egg whites. Drop by teaspoonful (walnut size) onto cookie sheet sprayed with nonstick spray. Bake at 350 degrees for 15 minutes. Makes 30 Servings.

SERVING SIZE - 2 COOKIES

Calories	45	Protein	1g
Total Fat	1g	Carbohydrate	9g
Saturated Fat	0g	Cholesterol	0mg
Sodium	8mg	Fiber	0g

EXCHANGES: 1/2 Starch

CHOCOLATE GINGER SPICE SQUARES

1. 1 Package Dry Gingerbread Mix
2. 2 Packages (3.4 oz.) Sugar Free Chocolate Fat Free Pudding Mix
   (not instant)
3. 1/4 Teaspoon Ground Cinnamon
4. 1 Cup Water

Combine above ingredients in a mixing bowl. Beat 1 minute on medium speed. Pour into 13x9x2-inch nonstick cake pan and bake at 350 degrees for 35 minutes. Allow to cool slightly or chill. Cut into squares. 32 Servings.

PER SERVING – ONE SQUARE

Calories	75	Protein	1g
Total Fat	2g	Carbohydrate	14g
Saturated Fat	0g	Cholesterol	0mg
Sodium	149mg	Fiber	0g

EXCHANGES: 1 Starch, 1/2 Fat

SNOW TOPPED BROWNIE MOUNDS

1. 1 Package Krusteaz Fat Free Brownie Mix
2. 1/3 Cup Water
3. 45 Miniature Marshmallows (about 1/2 cup)
4. 1 Teaspoon Cinnamon

Combine mix and water. It will be very stiff and sticky. When mix is thoroughly moistened, make small 1-inch balls. Place balls in mini muffin pans that have been sprayed with cooking spray. Push one minature marshmallow into each cookie ball. Bake at 350 degrees for 8-10 minutes. Makes 45 cookies.

PER SERVING – ONE COOKIE

Calories	49	Protein	0g
Total Fat	0g	Carbohydrate	10g
Saturated Fat	0g	Cholesterol	0mg
Sodium	36mg	Fiber	0g

EXCHANGES: 1/2 Starch

WALNUT/SPICE COOKIES

1. 1/4 Cup Sugar
2. 1 Teaspoon Pumpkin Pie Spice Seasoning
3. 1 Egg White (room temperature)
4. 1 Cup Walnuts (finely chopped)

Mix sugar and seasoning. Beat egg white on high for 1 minute. Gradually add sugar mixture. Beat until stiff. Fold in walnuts. Drop onto greased cookie sheet. Bake 35~40 minutes at 250 degrees.
12 Servings.

SERVING SIZE - 2 COOKIES

Calories	61	Protein	2g
Total Fat	4g	Carbohydrate	6g
Saturated Fat	0g	Cholesterol	0mg
Sodium	5mg	Fiber	0g

EXCHANGES: 1 Fat

SWEET CEREAL PUFFS

1. **3 Egg Whites**
2. **2/3 Cup Sugar**
3. **4 Cups Total Cereal**
4. **1/2 Cup Raisins**

Beat egg whites to a foam. Add sugar gradually, beating until stiff. Fold in cereal and raisins. Drop 2-inches apart on greased cookie sheet. Bake 14 minutes or until brown at 325 degrees. Cool.
20 Servings.

SERVING SIZE - 2 COOKIES

Calories	77	Protein	1g
Total Fat	0g	Carbohydrate	18g
Saturated Fat	0g	Cholesterol	0mg
Sodium	91mg	Fiber	1g

EXCHANGES: 1/2 Fruit, 1/2 Starch

FAT FREE CHERRY COBBLER

1. **2 Cans (16 oz.) Water Packed Sweet Cherries (drained, reserve juice)**
2. **1/2 Cup Self-Rising Flour**
3. **1/4 Cup Sugar**
4. **2/3 Cup Skim Milk**

Place cherries and 1/3 cup of the reserved juice in a 9-inch square pan. In a medium bowl, mix together flour, sugar and milk. Pour evenly over cherries. Bake uncovered at 350 degrees for 45 minutes.
6 Servings.

SERVING SIZE - 1/6 OF COBBLER

Calories	153	Protein	3g
Total Fat	0g	Carbohydrate	37g
Saturated Fat	0g	Cholesterol	0mg
Sodium	138mg	Fiber	2g

EXCHANGES: 1/2 Fruit, 1/2 Starch

LOW-FAT PINEAPPLE CAKE

1. **5 Egg Whites**
2. **1 Can (20 oz.) Water Packed Pineapple (crushed, drained)**
3. **1 Yellow Reduced Fat Cake Mix**
4. **1 Tablespoon Sugar**

Beat egg whites with electric mixer until foamy. Add drained pineapple and then cake mix. Spread mix in a floured 9x13 pan sprayed with nonstick spray. Sprinkle with sugar. Bake at 350 degrees for 35 minutes. 18 Servings.

SERVING SIZE - 1 SLICE

Calories	71	Protein	1g
Total Fat	1g	Carbohydrate	14g
Saturated Fat	0g	Cholesterol	0mg
Sodium	100mg	Fiber	0g

EXCHANGES: 1 Starch

CREAMY ORANGE CUPS

1. **2 Bananas**
2. **1 Can (6 oz.) Frozen Orange Juice**
3. **1/2 Cup Powdered Nonfat Milk**
4. **1 Cup Plain Yogurt**

In blender, puree bananas. Add remaining ingredients plus 1/2 cup water. Blend until foamy. Pour evenly into 6 small paper cups. Freeze. To eat, squeeze bottom of cup or serve with spoon.

SERVING SIZE - 1 CUP

Calories	120	Protein	5g
Total Fat	0g	Carbohydrate	26g
Saturated Fat	0g	Cholesterol	2mg
Sodium	59mg	Fiber	1g

EXCHANGES: 1/2 Milk, 1 1/2 Fruit

STRAWBERRY PINEAPPLE CUPS

1. 3 Ripe Bananas
2. 2 Containers (6 oz.) Fat Free Yogurt (any flavor)
3. 1 Package (10 oz.) Frozen Strawberries (thawed and undrained)
4. 1 Can (8 oz.) Crushed Pineapple (undrained, water packed)

Line 18 medium muffin cups with paper baking cups. In medium bowl, mash bananas with fork. Add remaining ingredients, stir until combined, spoon into cups. Freeze at least 3 hours or until firm. Remove from paper cups and let stand 10 minutes before serving. 18 Servings.

PER SERVING – ONE MUFFIN CUP

Calories	35	Protein	1g
Total Fat	0g	Carbohydrate	9g
Saturated Fat	0g	Cholesterol	0mg
Sodium	6mg	Fiber	1g

EXCHANGES: 1/2 Fruit

PINEAPPLE MELBA

1. 1 Fresh Pineapple (market sliced, 12 rings)
2. 3 Tablespoon Sugar
3. 1 Can (8 oz.) Sliced Peaches (drained, water packed)
4. 1/2 Cup Raspberries

Place pineapple rings on serving plate. Sprinkle with sugar. In blender, blend peaches until smooth. Top pineapple with peach sauce and fresh raspberries. 12 Servings.

PER SERVING – ONE RING

Calories	32	Protein	0g
Total Fat	0g	Carbohydrate	8g
Saturated Fat	0g	Cholesterol	0mg
Sodium	1mg	Fiber	1g

EXCHANGES: 1/2 Fruit

LOWFAT APPLESAUCE CAKE

1. **5 Egg Whites**
2. **2 1/2 Cups Unsweetened Applesauce**
3. **1 Yellow Reduced Fat Cake Mix**
4. **2 1/2 Tablespoons Sugar/Cinnamon Mix**

Beat egg whites with electric mixer until foamy. Mix in applesauce. Add cake mix and mix on medium speed for 1 minute. Spread mix in a 9x13 pan sprayed with nonstick spray and floured. Sprinkle cinnamon sugar mix on top. Bake at 350 degrees for 30 minutes. 18 Servings.

SERVING SIZE - 1/18 OF CAKE

Calories	248	Protein	1g
Total Fat	1g	Carbohydrate	59g
Saturated Fat	0g	Cholesterol	0mg
Sodium	101mg	Fiber	1g

EXCHANGES: 2 Starches, 2 Fruit

RICE PUDDING

1. **3 Cups Instant White Rice (cooked)**
2. **1 Cup Egg Beaters**
3. **1/3 Cup Sugar**
4. **3/4 Cup Skim Milk**

Mix all ingredients together. Place mixture in a 9-inch square pan that has been sprayed with nonstick spray. Bake at 325 degrees for 25 minutes. Serve warm or cold. 6 Servings.

SERVING SIZE - 1/2 CUP

Calories	171	Protein	6g
Total Fat	0g	Carbohydrate	35g
Saturated Fat	0g	Cholesterol	1mg
Sodium	73mg	Fiber	1g

EXCHANGES: 1/2 Very Lean Meat, 1 Starch

BLACK FOREST PUDDING

1. **1 Package Sugar Free Instant Chocolate Pudding Mix**
2. **1/2 Cup Plain Yogurt**
3. **1 Cup Skim Milk**
4. **1 Can (6 oz.) Sweet Cherries (chopped, liquid reserved)**

In large bowl, mix pudding mix, yogurt and milk. Add chopped cherries and 1/3 cup reserved cherry juice. Mix well and chill for at least 30 minutes.
4 Servings.

SERVING SIZE - 1/2 CUP

Calories	133	Protein	6g
Total Fat	1g	Carbohydrate	28g
Saturated Fat	0g	Cholesterol	2mg
Sodium	339mg	Fiber	0g

EXCHANGES: 1 Fruit, 1/2 Milk, 1/2 Starch

PUDDING SHAKE DESSERT

1. 1 Can (8 oz.) Water Packed Crushed Pineapple (undrained)
2. 1 1/2 Cup Skim Milk
3. 1 Small Box Sugar Free Vanilla Pudding

Place pineapple and juice in a 2-cup measuring cup. Add enough milk to fill 2 cups. Pour into a quart jar. Add pudding mix and cover tightly. Shake for 1 minute. Pour into serving bowl or individual dessert dishes. Chill at least 15 minutes before serving.
4 Servings.

SERVING SIZE - 1/2 CUP

Calories	72	Protein	3g
Total Fat	0g	Carbohydrate	14g
Saturated Fat	0g	Cholesterol	2mg
Sodium	186mg	Fiber	1g

EXCHANGES: 1/2 Milk, 1/2 Fruit

PUMPKIN YOGURT

1. 1 Can (16 oz.) Pumpkin
2. 2 Cups Plain Yogurt
3. 1/3 Cup Sugar
4. 2 Teaspoons Pumpkin Spice Mix

With electric mixer, mix above ingredients together and pour into a serving bowl. Chill at least one hour or overnight. 6 Servings.

SERVING SIZE - ONE

Calories	130	Protein	5g
Total Fat	0g	Carbohydrate	28g
Saturated Fat	0g	Cholesterol	2mg
Sodium	58mg	Fiber	21g

EXCHANGES: 1 Milk, 1 Starch

PEACH VANILLA SMOOTHIE

1. **1 Bag (16 oz.) Frozen Sliced Peaches (partially thawed)**
2. **1/3 Cup Brown Sugar**
3. **3/4 Cup Skim Milk**
4. **2 Teaspoons Vanilla Extract**

In food processor or blender, puree above ingredients. Can be served immediately or placed in freezer. If frozen, set out 30 minutes before serving. For creamier texture, whirl in food processor or blender before serving. 4 Servings.

SERVING SIZE - 1/4 MIXTURE

Calories	213	Protein	3g
Total Fat	0g	Carbohydrate	50g
Saturated Fat	0g	Cholesterol	1mg
Sodium	34mg	Fiber	3g

EXCHANGES: 2 Fruits

BANANAS ROSANNA

1. 1 Pint Fresh Strawberries
2. 1 Can (6 oz.) Orange Juice
   (concentrate, thawed, undiluted)
3. 3 Large Ripe Bananas (sliced)
4. 1 Carton (8 oz.) Fat Free Cool Whip

Wash, hull and cut up strawberries. Combine them in blender with undiluted orange juice concentrate and blend until smooth. Alternate banana slices with strawberry-orange sauce. Top with Cool Whip. Serve chilled. 8 Servings.

PER SERVING – 1/2 CUP

Calories	124	Protein	1g
Total Fat	1g	Carbohydrate	22g
Saturated Fat	0g	Cholesterol	1mg
Sodium	22mg	Fiber	1g

EXCHANGES: 1 1/2 Fruit

PINEAPPLE COCONUT SHERBET

1. 2 Cans (8 oz.) Unsweetened Crushed Pineapple (water packed, drained)
2. 2 Cups Nonfat Vanilla Yogurt
3. 1/2 Cup Unsweetened Shredded Coconut
4. 2 Tablespoons Honey

Combine all ingredients and stir well. Pour into shallow pan and freeze until partially set. Transfer to a bowl and beat 4 minutes. Pour into a container with cover and freeze until solid. Soften at room temperature for about 15 minutes before serving. 8 Servings.

PER SERVING – 1/2 CUP

Calories	60	Protein	1g
Total Fat	2g	Carbohydrate	10g
Saturated Fat	2g	Cholesterol	0mg
Sodium	20mg	Fiber	1g

EXCHANGES: 1/2 Fat, 1/2 Milk

SHERRIED FRUIT

1. 1 Package (12 oz.) Mixed Berries
2. 2 Cups Cantaloupe Balls
3. 1 Can (8 oz.) Pineapple Chunks (water packed)
4. 1/4 Cup Cooking Sherry

Combine fruit in large bowl. Add sherry and toss lightly. Cover and chill at least 2 hours or overnight. Served chilled. 6 Servings.

PER SERVING – 1/2 CUP

Calories	77	Protein	1g
Total Fat	0g	Carbohydrate	16g
Saturated Fat	0g	Cholesterol	0mg
Sodium	6mg	Fiber	3g

EXCHANGES: 1 Fruit

FROZEN BLUEBERRY-BANANA DESSERT

1. 2 Cups Fat Free Vanilla Frozen Yogurt
2. 2 Bananas
3. 1 Cup Frozen Blueberries
4. 1/4 Cup Frozen Concentrated Apple Juice

Thaw frozen yogurt just enough to cut into chunks. In blender, puree yogurt and remaining ingredients. Serve immediately or freeze for 15 minutes before serving. 6 Servings.

PER SERVING – 3/4 CUP

Calories	129	Protein	4g
Total Fat	0g	Carbohydrate	29g
Saturated Fat	0g	Cholesterol	2mg
Sodium	50mg	Fiber	1g

EXCHANGES: 1 Milk, 1 Fruit

CAPPUCCINO ICE

1. 3 Cups Strong Brewed Coffee
2. 2 Cups Lite Cool Whip (thawed)
3. 2 Tablespoons Sugar
4. 2 Tablespoons Cocoa

Combine all ingredients in blender. Blend at low speed until smooth. Pour into 8-inch square baking pan, cover and freeze until firm. Remove from freezer and let frozen mixture stand at room temperature for 30 minutes. Again spoon into blender and process until smooth. Return to baking pan, cover and freeze until firm. When ready to serve, let stand 5 minutes at room temperature and spoon into serving dishes. 6 Servings.

PER SERVING – 3/4 CUP

Calories	189	Protein	0g
Total Fat	10g	Carbohydrate	24g
Saturated Fat	0g	Cholesterol	2mg
Sodium	59mg	Fiber	0g

EXCHANGES: 1 1/2 Starch, 2 Fat

COMPANY PEACH DELIGHT

1. **2 Cans (16 oz.) Lite Peach Halves (water packed)**
2. **4 Tablespoons Fat Free Cream Cheese**
3. **6 Tablespoons Brown Sugar**
4. **1 Teaspoon Ground Cinnamon**

Fill center of peaches with 1 tablespoon cream cheese and place halves together. Combine brown sugar and cinnamon. Roll peaches in brown sugar mixture. Chill until ready to serve. 4 Servings.

PER SERVING – ONE PEACH

Calories	137	Protein	7g
Total Fat	0g	Carbohydrate	29g
Saturated Fat	0g	Cholesterol	5mg
Sodium	214mg	Fiber	1g

EXCHANGES: 1 Very Lean Meat, 1 1/2 Starch, 1/2 Fruit

CHOCOLATE MERINGUE BITES

1. 2 Egg Whites
2. 1/4 Teaspoons Cream of Tartar
3. 1/4 Cup Sugar
4. 1 Tablespoon Cocoa Powder

Beat egg whites and cream of tartar with electric mixer until white and glossy. Add sugar and cocoa and beat until stiff peaks form. Drop by heaping teaspoons onto a brown paper lined baking sheet. Bake 2 hours at 225 degrees. Turn oven off and leave meringues in oven for 2 more hours.
24 Servings.

SERVING SIZE - 2 BITES

Calories	14	Protein	0g
Total Fat	0g	Carbohydrate	3g
Saturated Fat	0g	Cholesterol	0mg
Sodium	5mg	Fiber	0g

EXCHANGES: Free Food for 2 'bites'

CHOCOLATE FUDGE PUDDING CAKE

1. 1 Box (8 oz.) Light Creamy Deluxe Fudge Brownie Mix
2. 1 Cup Skim Milk
3. 1/2 Cup Hot Water

Mix dry brownie mix and milk in a large bowl with electric mixer. Pour into a 9x13 pan sprayed with nonstick spray. Pour hot water over mixture and cut through with a knife. Bake uncovered at 350 degrees for 25 minutes. Do not overbake. 8 Servings.

SERVING SIZE - 1 SLICE

Calories	151	Protein	2g
Total Fat	6g	Carbohydrate	23g
Saturated Fat	1g	Cholesterol	1mg
Sodium	109mg	Fiber	0g

EXCHANGES: 1 Fat, 1 1/2 Starches

CREPES

1. **1 Cup Skim Milk**
2. **2 Egg Whites**
3. **3/4 Cup All Purpose Flour**
4. **1/8 Teaspoon Salt**

Place above ingredients in a blender. Blend until smooth. Pour batter into a bowl and cover. Chill at least 1 hour or overnight. Spray small skillet with nonstick cooking spray. Pour 1/4 cup batter into heated skillet. Cook over medium heat until bubbles form and it looks dry on top. Turn crepe over and cook on other side. Note - these cook very quickly. Serve warm. 8 Servings.

SERVING SIZE - 1 CREPE

Calories	58	Protein	3g
Total Fat	0g	Carbohydrate	11g
Saturated Fat	0g	Cholesterol	1mg
Sodium	243mg	Fiber	0g

EXCHANGES: 1/2 Starch

EASY BASIC GRAHAM CRACKER CRUST

1. 1 Box (12 oz.) Cinnamon Graham Crackers (1 1/2 cup crushed)
2. 1 Tablespoon Sugar
3. 1 Packet Size Equal Sugar Substitute
4. 1 1/2 Tablespoon Fat Free Margarine (melted)

Mix crushed graham crackers, sugars and melted margarine together until moist. Press into a pie pan that has been sprayed with a nonstick spray.
8 Servings.

SERVING SIZE - 1/8 PIE CRUST

Calories	191	Protein	3g
Total Fat	4g	Carbohydrate	35g
Saturated Fat	1g	Cholesterol	0mg
Sodium	272mg	Fiber	0g

EXCHANGES: 2 1/2 Starches, 1/2 Fat

FAT FREE PASTRY PIE CRUST

1. **1 Cup All Purpose Flour**
2. **3/4 Teaspoon Salt**
3. **4 Tablespoons Fat Free Margarine**
4. **3 Tablespoons Water**

Preheat oven to 475 degrees. With a fork mix together above ingredients until thoroughly mixed. Do not overwork dough. Shape this mixture into a ball and place between two pieces of waxed paper that has been dusted with flour. Roll dough into a circle large enough to fit into a 9-inch pie pan. Spray pan with nonstick spray and arrange crust centered in pan. Cut off any excess edges that hang over edge. Prick bottom of crust with fork and bake for 10 minutes or until golden brown. Cool before adding filling of your choice. 8 Servings.

SERVING SIZE - 1/8 PIE CRUST

Calories	59	Protein	2g
Total Fat	0g	Carbohydrate	12g
Saturated Fat	0g	Cholesterol	0mg
Sodium	245mg	Fiber	0g

EXCHANGES: 1 Starch

MERINGUE SHELL

1. 3 Egg Whites (room temperature)
2. 1/2 Cup Sugar

Preheat oven to 300 degrees. Spray a 9-inch pie pan with cooking spray. Beat egg whites until foamy. Gradually add sugar a tablespoon at a time and continue to beat until moist and stiff peaks form when beater is withdrawn. Spoon into pie pan so that it covers bottom and sides. Bake for 1 hour until light brown. Cool before filling shell. Good filled with fresh fruit. 8 Servings.

PER SERVING – ONE SLICE

Calories	63	Protein	1g
Total Fat	0g	Carbohydrate	14g
Saturated Fat	0g	Cholesterol	0mg
Sodium	21mg	Fiber	0g

EXCHANGES: 1 Starch

LOWFAT BAKED CUSTARD

1. 1 Can (12 0z.) Evaporated Skim Milk
2. 1/2 Teaspoon Vanilla
3. 3/4 Cup Egg Substitute
4. Sprinkle Nutmeg

Place milk in medium pan and heat until small bubbles form around edge. Mix eggs and vanilla in a bowl. Add 1 cup hot milk to egg mixture and blend. Return mixture back to remaining hot milk. Stir well. Heat, stirring constantly, until it almost simmers. Pour into 4 custard cups. Place cups in 1-inch of water in 9x13 pan. Sprinkle with nutmeg and bake at 325 degrees for 25 minutes. Chill 4 hours or overnight. 4 Servings.

SERVING SIZE - 1/2 CUP

Calories	182	Protein	14g
Total Fat	2g	Carbohydrate	27g
Saturated Fat	0g	Cholesterol	4mg
Sodium	210mg	Fiber	0g

EXCHANGES: 1 Milk, 1 Very Lean Meat

STRAWBERRY/BANANA PIE FILLING

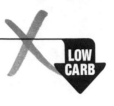

1. 1 Box (3 0z.) Sugar-Free Strawberry/Banana Jello
2. 2/3 Cup Boiling Water and 2 Cups Ice Cubes
3. 1 Carton (8oz.) Lite Cool Whip
4. 1 Cup Sliced Strawberries

Dissolve jello in boiling water. Stir jello about 3 minutes; add 2 cups ice cubes. Stir until ice melts and jello thickens. Blend Cool Whip into jello until smooth. Fold in strawberries. Chill until mixture will mound. Spoon into prepared pie crust. Refrigerate at 2 hours before serving. 8 Servings.

SERVING SIZE- 1/8 OF PIE (crust not included in analysis)

Calories	73	Protein	1g
Total Fat	4g	Carbohydrate	8g
Saturated Fat	0g	Cholesterol	1mg
Sodium	53 mg	Fiber	0g

EXCHANGES: 1/2 Fat, 1/2 Fruit

QUICK CHEESECAKE PIE

1. 1 Package (8 oz.) Fat Free Cream Cheese (softened)
2. 2 Cups Skim Milk
3. 1 Package Sugar Free Lemon Instant Fat Free Pudding Mix
4. 1 Reduced Fat Graham Cracker Pie Crust

Blend softened cream cheese and 1/2 cup of the milk. Add remaining milk and pudding mix. Beat slowly just until well mixed, about 1 minute...do not overbeat! Pour at once into graham cracker crust. Chill 1 hour. 8 Servings.

PER SERVING – ONE SLICE

Calories	173	Protein	9g
Total Fat	3g	Carbohydrate	22g
Saturated Fat	1g	Cholesterol	6mg
Sodium	438mg	Fiber	0g

EXCHANGES: 1/2 Milk, 1 1/2 Starch, 1 Meat

PEACH PIE

1. **7 Peaches (peeled, sliced)**
2. **1/4 Cup Sugar**
3. **2 Tablespoons Cornstarch**
4. **2 Tablespoons Low Fat Margarine**

Place all ingredients in pan and cook in saucepan on low to medium heat. Stir until sauce thickens. Refrigerate. Good served in meringue shell. 8 Servings.

PER SERVING – ONE SLICE

Calories	81	Protein	1g
Total Fat	1g	Carbohydrate	17g
Saturated Fat	0g	Cholesterol	0mg
Sodium	33mg	Fiber	1g

EXCHANGES: 1/2 Fruit, 1/2 Starch, 1/2 Fat

PEACH YOGURT PIE

1. 1 Can (8 3/4 oz.) Sliced Peaches (water packed)
2. 2 Containers (8 oz. each) Fat Free Fruit Flavored Yogurt
3. 1 Carton (8 oz.) Lite Cool Whip
4. 1 Reduced Fat Graham Cracker Crust

Combine fruit and yogurt, then fold in Cool Whip, blending well. Spoon into graham cracker crust. Freeze until firm, about 4 hours. Remove from freezer and place in refrigerator 30 minutes before serving. 8 Servings.

PER SERVING – ONE SLICE

Calories	230	Protein	3g
Total Fat	7g	Carbohydrate	33g
Saturated Fat	1g	Cholesterol	2mg
Sodium	189mg	Fiber	0g

EXCHANGES: 1 Milk, 2 Starches, 1 Fat

STRAWBERRY PIE

1. **1 Box (3 oz.) Sugar Free Strawberry Jello**
2. **1 Carton (8 oz.) Lite Cool Whip**
3. **1 Cup Sliced Strawberries**
4. **1 Reduced Fat Graham Cracker Crust**

Dissolve jello in 2/3 cup of boiling water. Stir jello about 3 minutes; add 2 cups ice cubes. Stir until ice melts and jello thickens. Blend Cool Whip into jello until smooth. Fold in strawberries. Chill until mixture will mound. Spoon into graham cracker crust. Refrigerate at least 2 hours before serving. 8 Servings.

PER SERVING – ONE SLICE

Calories	179	Protein	1g
Total Fat	7g	Carbohydrate	22g
Saturated Fat	1g	Cholesterol	1mg
Sodium	161mg	Fiber	0g

EXCHANGES: 1 1/2 Starches, 1 1/2 Fat

KOOLAIDE PIE

1. 1 Can (12 oz.) Skim Evaporated Milk (chilled)
2. 2/3 Cup Sugar
3. 1 Package (.15 oz.) Kool-Aid (any flavor)
4. 1 Reduced Fat Graham Cracker Crust

Beat milk until it is doubled in size. Add sugar and Kool-Aid and beat until thickened (about 5 minutes). Place in graham cracker crust and refrigerate until ready to serve. 8 Servings.

PER SERVING – ONE SLICE

Calories	234	Protein	5g
Total Fat	3g	Carbohydrate	41g
Saturated Fat	1g	Cholesterol	2mg
Sodium	191mg	Fiber	1g

EXCHANGES: 2 1/2 Starch, 1/2 Milk

BANANA CREAM PUDDING

1. 1 Package (.9 oz) Fat Free Sugar Free Jello Banana Cream Pudding Mix
2. 2 1/2 Cups Fat Free Milk
3. 12 Lowfat Vanilla Wafers
4. 2 Bananas (sliced)

Mix pudding with milk. Layer 6 cookies, 1 sliced banana and half of pudding. Repeat layers with remaining ingredients ending with pudding. Refrigerate. 6 Servings.

SERVING SIZE- 1/2 CUP

Calories	143	Protein	4g
Total Fat	3g	Carbohydrate	26g
Saturated Fat	1g	Cholesterol	2mg
Sodium	310 mg	Fiber	1g

EXCHANGES: 1/2 Fat, 1/2 Fruit

VANILLA SOUR CREAM PUDDING

1. 1 Cup Fat Free Sour Cream
2. 1 Cup Skim Milk
3. 1 Package (3 1/2 oz.) Sugar Free Vanilla Instant
   Fat Free Pudding
4. 1/2 Cup Low Fat Cool Whip

Combine sour cream and milk until smooth. Add
dry pudding mix and mix until smooth and slightly
thickened. Pour into serving dishes and top with
Cool Whip. 8 Servings.

PER SERVING - ONE

Calories	101	Protein	4g
Total Fat	2g	Carbohydrate	16g
Saturated Fat	0g	Cholesterol	1mg
Sodium	316mg	Fiber	0g

EXCHANGES: 1 Starch, 1 Fat, 1/2 Meat

PEACH CRISP

1. 2 Cans (16 oz.) Sliced Peaches (drained)
2. 1/4 Cup Sugar
3. 2 teaspoons Cornstarch
4. 3/4 Cup Lowfat Granola (without raisins)

In small bowl combine peaches, sugar and cornstarch. Spoon peach mixture into 4 custard cups coated with non-stick spray. Place cups on a baking sheet and sprinkle lowfat granola over tops of each custard cup. Bake at 400 degrees uncovered for 25 minutes or until thoroughly heated and tops are crisp. 4 Servings.

SERVING SIZE- 1/2 CUP

Calories	101	Protein	3g
Total Fat	3g	Carbohydrate	33g
Saturated Fat	1g	Cholesterol	0mg
Sodium	49 mg	Fiber	2g

EXCHANGES: 1 Starch, 1 Fruit, 1 Fat.

SWEET BERRY PUDDING

1. **1 Tablespoon Fat Free Margarine**
2. **1/2 of 16 oz. Loaf of French Bread (cut into 1/2 inch slices)**
3. **1 Package (16 oz.) Frozen Blackberries (thawed)**
4. **1/4 Cup Sugar**

Spread margarine on inside of a 10-cup metal mixing bowl. Line bottom and sides with bread slices. Bring berries, their juice and sugar to a boil in a heavy sauce pan over medium-high heat. Boil for 2 minutes. Lower heat and simmer 4 minutes longer. Spoon into bread lined bowl. Top berries with remaining bread slices. Cut away extra pieces of bread from sides of bowl. Top pudding with a piece of foil and a saucer. Weigh saucer down with a can of food or other heavy weight. Refrigerate 10 hours or overnight. Loosen edges with a table knife. Invert onto serving dish. Serve cold. 8 Servings.

SERVING SIZE - ONE

Calories	136	Protein	3g
Total Fat	1g	Carbohydrate	29g
Saturated Fat	0g	Cholesterol	0mg
Sodium	154mg	Fiber	4g

EXCHANGES: 1/2 Fruit, 1 Starch

INDEX

APPETIZERS

Almond Delight Dip, 21
Almond Fruit Dip, 23
Apple Curry Dip, 24
Artichoke Ranch Dip, 42
Avocado and Leek Dip, 40
Bagel Chips, 54
California Dip, 33
Caramel Fruit Dip, 22
Chile Salsa, 28
Chili Con Queso, 27
Cottage Cheese-Cucumber
  Spread, 9
Cottage Cheese Dip, 34
Crab Delight, 50
Cream Cheese Dip, 37
Creamy Dill Dip, 36
Curry Dip, 44
Dill Dip, 35
Easy Crab Spread, 5
Fresh Strawberry Dip, 20
Fruited Cheese Spread, 25
Green Chili Pie, 8
Ham and Pimiento Spread, 10
Hidden Valley Ranch Cheese
  Puffs, 47
Homemade Fat Free Tortilla
  Chips, 53
Hot Artichoke Dip, 6
Hot Artichoke Spread, 13
Hot Seafood Dip, 6
Italian Shrimp Dip, 4
Jalapeno Pie, 7
Light Guacamole, 51
Mexican Avocado Dip, 29
Mexican Meatballs, 30
Mini Quiches, 18
Party Drummettes, 32
Party Rye Bread, 12
Pimiento Cheese Spread I, 15

Pimiento Cheese Spread II, 16
Pineapple Ball, 19
Pizza Crackers, 52
Potato Skins, 46
Roquefort Dip, 45
San Antone Bean Dip, 17
Sherried Meatballs, 31
Shrimp Spread, 3
Sour Cream Dip, 37
Spanish Olive Spread, 14
Spring Vegetable Dip, 38
Stuffed Mushrooms, 11
Tangy Dip, 43
Tomato Sour Cream Dip, 41
Tortilla Rollups, 49
Tropical Cheese Spread, 26
Veggie Dippin Dip, 48

BEEF

BBQ Cups, 294
Beef Goulash, 287
Beef Stroganoff, 278
Broiled Flank Steak, 291
Cabbage and Beef Dish, 284
Chili Meal Loaf, 280
Company Beef Tenderloin, 274
Coney Island Burgers, 271
Creole Pepper Steak, 272
Flank Steak, 292
Flank Steak and Spinach
  Pinwheels, 288
Flank Steak Joy, 290
Ground Meat and Bean
  Casserole, 282
Indian Corn, 293
Meat and Potato Dinner, 285
Mexican Meatloaf, 281
Mustard Onion Chuck Roast,
  276
New York Roast Beef, 295

Orange Pepper Steak, 273
Round Steak Bake, 277
Salisbury Steak, 283
Savory Sunday Roast, 296
Sherried Beef, 289
Spanish Hamburgers, 279
Stuffed Bell Peppers, 297
Swiss Steak, 275
Tator Tot Casserole, 298
Vegetable Meat Dish, 286

BREADS
Bagel Chips, 54
Crepes, 362
Homemade Fat Free Tortilla
   Chips, 53
Party Rye Bread, 12
Pizza Crackers, 52

CAKES
Angel Cake, 335
Chocolate Fudge Pudding Cake,
   361
Low Fat Applesauce Cake, 348
Low Fat Pineapple Cake, 344

CHEESE
Chili Con Queso, 27
Creamy Cheesy Pasta, 309
Jalapeno Pie, 7
Mini Quiches, 18

CHICKEN
Apricot Lemon Chicken, 176
Baked Chicken Parmesan, 192
Baked Chimichanges, 161
Broiled and Spicy Chicken, 196
Cajun Chicken, 183
Cherry Chicken, 164
Chicken and Rice, 202

Chicken and Rice Deluxe, 181
Chicken Asparagus Rolls, 165
Chicken Breast with
   Mushrooms, 198
Chicken Cacciatore, 194
Chicken Dijon, 190
Chicken Marsala, 173
Chicken Sour Cream, 168
Chicken With A Glaze, 188
Company Chicken, 191
Confetti Chicken, 195
Crock Pot Chicken, 167
Crunchy Cornflake Chicken,
   184
Fiesta Chicken, 170
Honey Chicken, 199
Honey Mustard Chicken, 187
Italian Chicken, 201
Italian Mushroom Chicken, 171
Lemonade Chicken, 178
Lemon Garlic Chicken, 197
Lemon Pepper Chicken, 193
Lime Chicken, 174
Mexican Chicken, 200
Mexican Chicken II, 166
Mushroom Chicken, 179
Onion Ring Chicken, 172
Open Faced Chicken Cordon
   Bleu, 175
Orange Chicken, 162
Oven Barbecued Chicken, 189
Oven Fried Chicken, 186
Parmesan Chicken, 180
Savory Baked Lemon Chicken,
   163
Spicy Tomato Chicken, 182
Sweet Orange Chicken, 177
Tangy Chicken, 169
Tasty Chicken, 203
Tarragon Chicken, 160

Yogurt Cumin Chicken, 159
Zesty Crisp Chicken, 185

COOKIES
Chocolate Ginger Spice
  Squares, 339
Chocolate Meringue Bites, 360
Oatmeal Macaroons, 338
Orange Coconut Balls, 331
Raisin Treats, 332
Snow Topped Brownie Mounds,
  340
Sweet Cereal Puffs, 342
Walnut Spice Cookies, 341

DESSERTS
(see Cakes, Cookies, Pies,
Puddings, and Desserts, Other)

DESSERTS, OTHER
Bananas Rosenna, 354
Black Forest Pudding, 350
Cappuccino Ice, 358
Cherry Vanilla Trifle, 330
Company Peach Delight, 359
Creamy Orange Cups, 345
Crepes, 362
Frozen Blueberry-Banana
  Dessert, 357
Gingerale Baked Apples, 337
Gingersnap Baked Pears, 336
Low Fat Baked Custard, 366
Peach Crisp, 375
Peach Vanilla Smoothie, 353
Pineapple Melba, 347
Pineapple Coconut Sherbert,
  355
Pineapple Orange Fluff, 333
Pudding Shake Dessert, 351
Pumpkin Yogurt, 352

Sherried Fruit, 356
Strawberry Pineapple Cups, 346
Strawberry Trifle, 329

DIPS
Almond Delight Dip, 21
Almond Fruit Dip, 23
Apple Curry Dip, 24
Artichoke Ranch Dip, 42
Avocado and Leek Dip, 40
California Dip, 33
Caramel Fruit Dip, 22
Chili Salsa, 28
Cottage Cheese Dip, 34
Cream Cheese Dip, 37
Creamy Dill Dip, 36
Curry Dip, 44
Dill Dip, 35
Fresh Strawberry Dip, 20
Hot Seafood Dip, 6
Italian Shrimp Dip, 5
Light Guacamole, 51
Mexican Avocado Dip, 29
Roquefort Dip, 45
San Antone Bean Dip, 17
Spring Vegetable Dip, 39
Tangy Dip, 43
Tomato Sour Cream Dip,
Veggie Dippin Dip, 48

FISH
Baked Cod Vinaigrette, 212
Baked Orange Roughy, 214
Broiled Cod, 211
Broiled Salmon Steaks, 224
Broiled Shrimp, 209
Company Halibut Fillets, 218
Crispy Baked Fish, 241
Crunchy Baked Fish, 239
Dijon Salmon, 237

Dill Fillets, 227
Easy Cheesy Fish Fillets, 216
Fish Delight, 215
Fish With Lime, 228
Garlic Snapper, 233
Gazpacho Fillets, 231
Grilled Tuna Steaks, 234
Herbed Salmon Steaks, 238
Italian Fish Fillets, 232
Lemon Butter Dill Fish, 223
Marinated Grilled Shrimp, 210
Orange Roughy With Red
    Peppers, 217
Parmesan Fillets, 229
Party Baked Fish, 240
Quick Crab Stir Fry, 242
Scallop Kabobs, 235
Seasoned Orange Roughy, 236
Shrimp Kabobs, 220
Shrimp Marinara, 207
Spanish Fish, 213
Spicy Baked Fillets, 225
Stuffed Fish Fillets, 230
Sweet Mustard Fish, 219
Sweet Orange Fillets, 226
Tangy Apricot Fish, 222
Tarragon Fish, 221
Texas Boiled Beer Shrimp, 208

PASTA
Creamy Cheesy Pasta, 309
Garlic Pasta Primavera, 301
Herbed Pasta, 303
Italian Chicken Pasta, 310
Lemon Pasta, 304
Mamma Mia Pasta, 302
Pasta Primavera With
    Parmesan, 305
Pasta Salad, 68
Pasta With Spicy Clam Sauce,
308
Seafood Pasta, 306
Veggie Pasta Bake, 307

PIES
Easy Basic Graham Cracker
    Crust, 363
Fat Free Cherry Cobbler, 343
Fat Free Pastry Pie Crust, 364
Koolaide Pie, 372
Meringue Shell, 365
Peach Pie, 369
Peach Yogurt Pie, 370
Quick Cheese Cake Pie, 368
Strawberry Banana Pie Filling,
    367
Strawberry Peach Yogurt Pie,
334
Strawberry Pie, 371

PORK
Baked Pork Tenderloin, 253
Best Pork Tenderloin, 250
Deviled Pork Roast, 257
Hawaiian Baked Pork, 263
Honey Mustard Pork
    Tenderloin, 252
Lemon Garlic Roast Pork, 260
Marinated Pork Tenderloin, 251
Mustard-Apricot Pork Chops,
247
Orange Pork Chops, 249
Peachy Pork, 264
Pineapple Pork, 254
Polynesian Pork, 266
Pork Casserole, 267
Pork Chops With Red Cabbage,
246
Pork Stir Fry, 265
Pork Tenderloin Supreme, 258

Quickie Hawaiian Pork, 261
Raisin Spiced Pork Chops, 255
Roast Pork in Marinade, 262
Sage Seasoned Pork Loins, 259
Saucy Pork Chops, 256
Savory Broiled Pork Chops, 248
Tex Mex Chops, 245

POTATOES
Chili-Baked Fries, 114
Cottage Cheese Stuffed Baked Potatoes, 110
Cottaged Sweet Potatoes, 111
Gingered Sweet Potatoes, 112
Herbed New Potatoes, 105
Mashed Potatoes and Carrots, 109
New Potato Vinaigrette, 104
Potato Skins, 46
Potatoes O'Brien, 106
Roasted New Potatoes, 107
Scalloped Potatoes, 113
Spicy New Potatoes, 108
Stuffed Bake Potatoes, 103
Sweet Potato Salad, 59

PUDDINGS
Banana Cream Pudding, 373
Black Forest Pudding, 350
Chocolate Fudge Pudding, Cake, 361
Low Fat Baked Custard, 366
Pudding Shake Dessert, 351
Rice Pudding, 349
Sweet Berry Pudding, 376
Vanilla Sour Cream Pudding, 374

SALADS
Apple Coleslaw, 60
Apple Salad With Feta Cheese, 94
Beet and Onion Salad, 75
Bell Pepper Salad, 61
Broccoli Salad, 76

Carrot Raisin Celery Salad, 67
Carrot Salad, 66
Corn Salad, 78
Cucumber Salad, 79
Cucumber Strawberry Salad, 65
Frozen Pineapple Cranberry Salad, 91
Fruit and Spinach Salad, 89
Green Bean Salad, 74
Green Bean and Baby Corn Salad, 82
Hearts of Palm Salad, 62
Hearty Spinach and Mushroom Salad, 85
Honey Cucumber Salad, 80
Italian Tomato Cheese Salad, 64
Layered Fruit Salad, 95
Luncheon Tuna Salad, 58
Mandarin Salad, 96
Marinated Cauliflower Salad, 77
Marinated Vegetable Salad, 57
Mushroom Salad, 98
Orange Salad, 70
Orange Juice Dressing, 97
Pasta Salad, 68
Pea Salad, 92
Quick Melon Salad, 99
Romaine Strawberry Salad, 90
Seafood Pasta Salad, 69
Seafood Salad, 71
Snow Pea Salad, 63
Spinach Chicken Salad, 73
Spinach Salad, 84
Spinach With Sprouts, 88
Sunny Spinach Salad, 83
Sunshine Salad, 86
Sweet and Sour Cucumber Salad, 81
Sweet Potato Salad, 59
Tangy Spinach Salad, 87
Turkey Salad, 72
Waldorf Salad, 93

SAUCES

Basic White Sauce, 320
Chicken Gravy, 315
Chocolate Sauce, 313
Four Minute Gravy, 323
Garlic Tomato Mayonnaise, 318
Green Chile Sauce, 314
Mock Mayonnaise Spread, 319
Orange Cream Cheese Glaze, 324
Quick Hollandaise Sauce, 317
Spicy Topper, 322
Strawberry Sauce, 325
Tangy Sour Cream, 321
Zippy Fruit Sauce, 316

SPREADS

Cottage Cheese-Cucumber Spread, 9
Easy Crab Spread, 5
Fruited Cheese Spread, 25
Ham and Pimiento Spread, 10
Hot Artichoke Spread, 13
Pimiento Cheese Spread I, 15
Pimiento Cheese Spread II, 16
Pineapple Ball, 19
Shrimp Spread, 3
Spanish Olive Spread, 14
Tropical Cheese Spread, 26

VEGETABLES

Asparagus In Lemon Butter, 138
Asparagus With Sesame Seeds, 141
Baked Onion Rings, 129
Braised Celery, 156
Candied Acorn Squash, 118
Carrot Casserole I, 152
Carrot Casserole II, 153
Carrots and Zucchini, 155
Cheesy Cauliflower, 134
Chili-Baked Fries, 114
Cold Vegetable Dish, 127

Corn Relish, 143
Cottage Cheese Stuffed Baked Potatoes, 110
Cottaged Sweet Potatoes, 111
Dijon Broccoli, 132
French Onion Rings, 142
Garlic Green Beans, 116
Ginger Carrots, 150
Gingered Sweet Potatoes, 112
Green Beans With Dill, 117
Herbed New Potatoes, 105
Herb Tomato Slices, 126
Hot Cabbage, 136
Italian Eggplant, 115
Italian Style Broccoli, 131
Lemon Asparagus and Baby Carrots, 139
Lemon Brussel Sprouts, 135
Marinated Vegetables, 128
Marvelous Mushrooms, 146
Mashed Potatoes and Carrots, 109
Minted Carrots, 154
New Potatoes Vinaigrette, 104
Okra Succotash, 137
Parmesan Broccoli and Mushrooms, 133
Peachy Carrots, 151
Potatoes O'Brien, 106
Roasted New Potatoes, 107
Sauteed Broccoli, 130
Sauteed Spinach, 123
Scalloped Potatoes, 113
Sesame Rice, 121
Sesame Snow Peas, 148
Skillet Squash, 119
Snow Peas and Mushrooms, 149
Southwestern Corn, 144
Spicy Corn Bake, 145
Spicy New Potatoes, 108
Spinach Casserole, 122
Spinach Topped Tomatoes, 124
Stuffed Baked Potatoes, 103
Tangy Italian Mushrooms, 147

Tarragon Asparagus, 140
Tomato Stack, 125
Zucchini Squash, 120

For Additional Copies...

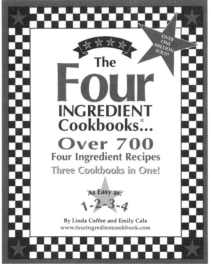

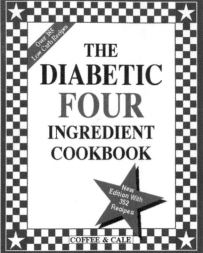

Please send me...

_____ copies of *The Four Ingredient Cookbooks* @ $19.95 each	$_____
_____ copies of *The Diabetic Four Ingredient Cookbook* @ $19.95 each	$_____
Postage & handling @ $3.50 each	$_____
Sub-Total	$_____
Texas residents add 8.25% sales tax per book @ $1.93 each	$_____
Canadian orders add additional $6.60 per book	$_____
Total Enclosed	$_____

❑ Check enclosed made payable to "Coffee and Cale"

Or charge to my

❑ VISA   ❑ MasterCard   ❑ Discover   *(Canada - credit card only)*

Card # _____   Exp. Date _____

Ship to:

Name_____

Address _____Apt.# _____

City _____ State _____ Zip _____

E-mail address _____

Phone _____
(Must have for Credit Card Orders)

Coffee & Cale
P.O. Box 2121 • Kerrville, TX 78029 • 1-800-757-0838
www.fouringredientcookbook.com • email:areglen@ktc.com
For Wholesale Information: • (830) 895-5528

Also Available

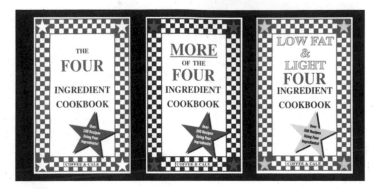

Our *original* soft cover cookbooks!

___ copies of *The Four Ingredient Cookbook* @ $12.90 each $_____

___ copies of *More of the Four Ingredient Cookbook* @ $12.90 each $_____

___ copies of *Low-Fat & Light Four Ingredient Cookbook* @ $12.90 each $_____

Special Savings!!!

Buy any 3 original soft cover cookbooks for only $23.50!!! $_____

above prices include shipping & handling of $2.95 per book

Texas residents add 8.25% sales tax $_____

Canadian orders add additional $3.30 per book $_____

Total Enclosed $_____

❏ Check enclosed made payable to "Coffee and Cale"

Or charge to my

❏ VISA   ❏ MasterCard   ❏ Discover   *(Canada - credit card only)*

Card #_____ Exp. Date_____

Ship to:

Name _____

Address_____Apt.#_____

City _____ State _____ Zip_____

E-mail address _____

Phone_____

(Must have for Credit Card Orders)

Coffee & Cale

P.O. Box 2121 • Kerrville, TX 78029 • 1-800-757-0838

www.fouringredientcookbook.com • email:areglen@ktc.com

For Wholesale Information: • (830) 895-5528